A
CROHN'S DISEASE COOKBOOK

75 Healing Recipes, healthy treats for nourishing your body and relieving Symptoms in the management of Inflammatory Bowel Disease

A 14 days meal plan to get you started

Katherine C. Collins

COPYRIGHT

Copyright © 2024 by Katherine C. Collins
All rights reserved. Without the prior written permission of the author, no part of this book may be reproduced, distributed, or transmitted in any form or by any means, including photocopying, recording, or other electronic or mechanical methods except in the case of brief quotations embodied in critical reviews and certain other noncommercial uses permitted by copyright law.

DISCLAIMER:

The information contained in this book is for educational and informational purposes only. The author and publisher of this book are not trained medical professionals, and the information provided is not intended to be a substitute for professional medical advice, diagnosis, or treatment that is offered by a qualified medical professional. In the event that you have any inquiries about a medical problem, you should always consult with your primary care physician or another trained health expert.

The author and publisher of this book make no representations or warranties with respect to the accuracy, applicability, fitness, or completeness of the contents of this book. They expressly disclaim all warranties, whether explicit or implied, as well as any claims about merchantability or suitability for any particular purpose. In the event that any loss or damage occurs as a result of the utilization of or reliance on the information not included in this book, the author nor the publisher shall not be deemed responsible. Readers should conduct their own research and exercise their own judgment when making decisions related to their health, diet, exercise, or any other matters discussed in this book.

By reading this book, you agree to indemnify and keep harmless the author and publisher from and against any losses, claims, damages, obligations, and costs resulting from or connected to your use or misuse of the material included herein.

Your use of this book acknowledges your agreement of these terms and conditions. If you do not agree with these terms, you should not use this book.

Thank you for respecting the intellectual property rights and disclaimer provided herein.

Here is the Bonus

A 14 days meal plan to get you started

✦ Day 1:

Breakfast: Banana Oatmeal Breakfast Bowl
Lunch: Quinoa Salad with Grilled Chicken
Dinner: Baked Salmon with Roasted Vegetables
Snack: Almond Butter Energy Balls

✦ Day 2:

Breakfast: Scrambled Eggs with Spinach
Lunch: Chickpea Salad Sandwich
Dinner: Vegan Lentil Curry
Snack: Greek Yogurt with Honey and Nuts

✦ Day 3:

Breakfast: Greek Yogurt Parfait
Lunch: Stuffed Bell Peppers with Ground Turkey
Dinner: Quinoa Buddha Bowl
Snack: Carrot Cake Smoothie

✦ Day 4:

Breakfast: Smoothie Bowl
Lunch: Vegan Pasta Primavera
Dinner: Baked Chicken Breast with Sweet Potato Mash
Snack: Frozen Grapes

✦ Day 5:

Breakfast: Chia Seed Pudding
Lunch: Vegan Lentil Soup
Dinner: Spaghetti Squash with Tomato Basil Sauce
Snack: Coconut Yogurt Parfait

✦ Day 6:

Breakfast: Rice Cake with Peanut Butter
Lunch: Sweet Potato and Black Bean Tacos
Dinner: Mushroom and Spinach Risotto
Snack: Almond Joy Smoothie

✦ Day 7:

Breakfast: Sautéed Vegetable Omelette
Lunch: Vegetable and Lentil Soup
Dinner: Tofu Stir-Fry with Brown Rice
Snack: Frozen Banana Bites

✦ Day 8:

Breakfast: Overnight Oats
Lunch: Spinach and Feta Turkey Burgers
Dinner: Vegetable and Lentil Curry
Snack: Chocolate Covered Strawberries

✦ Day 9:

Breakfast: Avocado Toast
Lunch: Quinoa and Vegetable Salad
Dinner: Eggplant Parmesan
Snack: Berry Smoothie

⁜ Day 10:

Breakfast: Frittata Muffins
Lunch: Mediterranean Chickpea Salad
Dinner: Lemon Herb Grilled Chicken with Roasted Vegetables
Snack: Peanut Butter Banana Smoothie

⁜ Day 11:

Breakfast: Rice Porridge
Lunch: Tofu Stir-Fry with Brown Rice
Dinner: Baked Salmon with Quinoa Salad
Snack: Pumpkin Chia Seed Pudding

⁜ Day 12:

Breakfast: Coconut Flour Pancakes
Lunch: Vegan Burrito Bowl
Dinner: Grilled Steak with Roasted Asparagus
Snack: Greek Yogurt with Berries

⁜ Day 13:

Breakfast: Mixed Greens Salad
Lunch: Vegetable and Quinoa Stuffed Portobello Mushrooms
Dinner: Mushroom and Spinach Risotto
Snack: Almond Butter Energy Balls

⁜ Day 14:

Breakfast: Banana "Nice" Cream
Lunch: Quinoa and Vegetable Salad
Dinner: Vegan Lentil Shepherd's Pie
Snack: Frozen Grapes

ABOUT THE AUTHOR

Katherine C. Collins is a passionate cook with a profound interest in healthy eating and culinary discovery. Her adventure in the world of food started at an early age, inspired by a desire for ingredients, tastes, and ethnic cuisines. With years of expertise in the culinary arts, Katherine has perfected her talents in preparing tasty and healthy meals that feed the body and thrill the palette. Driven by a passion for health and wellbeing, Katherine went on a personal mission to understand the tremendous influence of food on total well-being. Inspired by the transformational potential of nutritious foods and mindful cooking habits, she went on a quest to share her expertise and love for healthier living with others.

As a committed wife and cook, Katherine recognizes the significance of maintaining a supportive and healthy atmosphere at home. Together with her husband, she explores the unlimited possibilities of producing healthful and delectable meals that provide pleasure and life to their lives.

Katherine's cooking concept is centered on simplicity, harmony, and originality. She believes in the power of food to heal, invigorate, and connect individuals to their bodies and the world around them. Through her work, Katherine strives to inspire and motivate people to adopt a lifestyle of nutritious eating, thoughtful living, and culinary discovery.

When she's not experimenting in the kitchen or sharing her culinary ideas, Katherine likes spending time outdoors, practicing yoga, and appreciating moments of quiet meditation with her loved ones. She is devoted to living with purpose, gratitude, and a profound appreciation for the multitude of tastes and experiences that life has to offer.

TABLE OF CONTENTS

INTRODUCTION:

Welcome to the "Crohn's Disease Cookbook: Your Culinary Guide to Managing Crohn's Disease." Inside this guide, you'll go on a trip where delicious tastes and healthy eating meets, offering tasty recipes and important insights into beating Crohn's disease with food. Imagine a life where each meal isn't just about eating but also about helping you beat Crohn's disease. For millions worldwide, living with this condition means facing random signs like stomach pain, diarrhea, tiredness, and starvation. But within these difficulties, there's hope: the power of a carefully planned diet.

As a professional cook with a deep-rooted love for fitness, I've experienced directly the powerful effect that food can have on our health and well-being. Through careful study and cooperation with healthcare experts, I've created this recipe as a complete resource for people managing the difficulties of Crohn's disease. This book is more than just a collection of recipes—it's a testament to the resilience of the human spirit and the endless possibilities of cooking creativity. Within these pages, you'll find a great trove of healthy meals meant to support your journey to wellness. From bright salads and warm soups to filling mains and delicious desserts, each recipe is thoughtfully selected to provide a symphony of flavors and important nutrients.

Yet, beyond the world of tempting taste buds, this recipe serves as a light of knowledge, giving important insights into the science behind Crohn's disease and the key role that food plays in its management. You'll find practical tips for building a Crohn's-friendly kitchen, strategies for improving nutrition without losing taste, and advice on handling common dietary mistakes. Above all, this recipe is an ode to the power of community and shared experience. Within its pages, you'll find comfort in knowing that you're not alone on this trip.
Whether you're a seasoned cook or a beginner in the kitchen, whether you've just been diagnosed or have been living with Crohn's disease for years, this book is your friend, your ally, and your guide to taking control of your health and your life.

So, let's start on this cooking trip together—a journey where food is not just survival but a source of healing, hope, and joy. With each dish, may you find food for your body, comfort for your soul, and inspiration for a life lived to the fullest.

UNDERSTANDING CROHN'S DISEASE

What is Crohn's Disease? Crohn's disease is a chronic inflammatory condition that mainly affects the digestive tract, although it can involve any part of the gastrointestinal (GI) tract from the mouth to the anus. It is marked by inflammation of the walls of the digestive system, which can lead to a range of symptoms and problems. The exact cause of Crohn's disease is not fully known, but it is thought to involve a mix of genetic, environmental, and immune system factors. The immune system, which usually guards the body from illness and disease, may mistakenly attack the healthy cells of the digestive tract, leading to inflammation. Crohn's disease is a chronic condition, meaning that it tends to be life long and can flare up regularly. These flare-ups may be caused by different factors such as stress, food, medicines, or other underlying health problems.

Complications of Crohn's disease may include intestinal strictures (narrowing of the intestines), fistulas (abnormal links between different parts of the intestines or between the intestines and other organs), sores, malnutrition, and a higher risk of colon cancer.

Treatment for Crohn's disease aims to lower inflammation, improve symptoms, and avoid consequences. This may involve medicines such as anti-inflammatory drugs, immunosuppressants, biologics, antibiotics, and symptom-relieving medications. In some cases, surgery may be necessary to remove damaged parts of the digestive system or fix problems such as fistulas or strictures. Additionally, lifestyle improvements such as food changes, stress management, regular exercise, and smoking quitting may help control symptoms and improve general quality of life for people with Crohn's disease.

FACTORS OF CROHN'S DISEASE:

Causes and Risk: The exact cause of Crohn's disease is not fully known, but it is thought to involve a mix of genetic, environmental, and immune system factors.

Here's a breakdown of the possible reasons and risk factors related with Crohn's disease:
* Genetics
* Immune system dysfunction
* Environmental factors
* Smoking
* Age and ethnicity
* Geographic location
* Dietary factors

Symptoms: Crohn's disease can appear with a range of symptoms, which may vary in intensity and can affect any part of the gastrointestinal system. Common signs include:
* Persistent Diarrhea
* Stomach Pain and Cramping
* Tiredness
* Weight Loss
* Fever
* Rectal Bleeding
* Loss of hunger
* Nutritional shortages
* Joint Pain
* Skin Problems
* Eye Problems
* Mouth Ulcers

Diagnosis: Diagnosing Crohn's disease usually involves a mix of medical history, physical examination, blood tests, imaging studies, and surgical treatments. The testing process may include:
* Medical History and Physical Examination
* Blood Tests
* Stool Tests
* Imaging Studies
* Endoscopic Procedures
* Biopsy

The evaluation of Crohn's disease can be complicated and may require teamwork between healthcare workers, including gastroenterologists, radiologists, pathologists, and other experts. Early detection and treatment are important for successfully treating Crohn's disease and minimizing problems. If you think you may have Crohn's disease or are having signs suggestive of the condition, it's important to speak with a healthcare provider for evaluation and proper treatment.

Impact on Daily Life: Living with Crohn's disease can have a deep effect on various parts of daily life, ranging from physical health and mental well-being to social relationships and general quality of life. Here are some ways in which Crohn's disease can affect daily life:

* Physical Symptoms
* Nutritional Concerns
* Medicine Management
* Emotional Well-being
* Social Isolation
* Work and School
* Financial Burden

Despite these difficulties, many people with Crohn's disease find ways to adapt, deal, and thrive with the help of healthcare workers, family, friends, and community resources. Seeking effective treatment, adopting healthy living habits, learning stress management techniques, and connecting with others who share similar experiences can help people handle the impact of Crohn's disease on daily life and achieve a better quality of life.

THE ROLE OF NUTRITION IN MANAGING CROHN'S DISEASE

Nutrition plays a key role in controlling Crohn's disease. While food alone cannot fix Crohn's disease, making informed dietary choices can help lessen symptoms, reduce inflammation, promote healing, and improve general well-being.

Here's a thorough look at the role of diet in controlling Crohn's disease:

Symptom Management: Certain foods and eating patterns can cause or worsen signs of Crohn's disease, such as stomach pain, diarrhea, and bloating. By finding and avoiding trigger items, people can reduce disease flare-ups and improve their quality of life.

Nutrient Absorption: Inflammation and damage to the bowels in Crohn's disease can impair the intake of nutrients, leading to deficiencies in vitamins, minerals, and other important nutrients. Optimal diet is important for keeping general health, supporting immune function, and promoting healing of the gut walls.

Maintaining Adequate Nutrition: Individuals with Crohn's disease may experience lower hunger, dietary limits, and problems handling certain foods, which can make it challenging to meet their nutritional needs. Ensuring an adequate amount of calories, protein, vitamins, and minerals is important for avoiding starvation and supporting general health.

Balanced Diet: A well-balanced diet that includes a range of nutrient-dense foods is suggested for people with Crohn's disease. Emphasizing whole foods such as fruits, veggies, whole grains, lean meats, and healthy fats can provide necessary nutrients while reducing the intake of processed foods, sugary sugars, and fatty fats.

Hydration: Chronic diarrhea and higher fluid loses linked with Crohn's disease can lead to dehydration and chemical issues. Staying hydrated by drinking plenty of fluids, including water, herbal teas, and electrolyte-rich drinks, is important for keeping hydration and supporting gut health.

Fiber Intake: Dietary fiber can be helpful for gut health, but some people with Crohn's disease may have trouble handling high-fiber foods, especially during flare-ups. Gradually increasing fiber intake and picking easily digestible forms of fiber, such as cooked veggies and soluble fiber sources like oats and psyllium, may help promote regularity and improve gut health.

Special Diets: Some people with Crohn's disease may benefit from special food methods suited to their unique needs and tastes. These may include the low-FODMAP diet, which restricts certain types of carbohydrates that can react in the gut and cause stomach complaints, or the specific carbohydrate diet (SCD), which removes complex carbohydrates and focuses on easily digested foods.

Supplementation: In some cases, food supplements may be suggested to address specific nutritional deficits or support gut health. These may include vitamin and mineral pills, probiotics, omega-3 fatty acids, and other specific nutritional treatments.

Individualized Approach: The treatment of Crohn's disease through nutrition should be highly individualized, taking into account factors such as disease intensity, symptoms, dietary limits, food allergies, and personal tastes. Working closely with a qualified dietitian or healthcare provider can help people create a personalized nutrition plan that meets their unique needs and goals.

IMPORTANCE OF DIET IN CROHN'S DISEASE MANAGEMENT

Here's a list of the role of food in Crohn's disease management:
*It helps in reducing inflammations
*It provides nutritional Support
*It provides a balance in Gut Microbiota
*It provides strategies in managing symptoms such as:
-Low-FODMAP Diet: Restricts certain types of carbs that can react in the gut and cause stomach complaints such as gas, bloating, and diarrhea. This diet may be helpful for people with Crohn's disease who experience symptoms linked to carbohydrate loss.
-Specific Carbohydrate Diet (SCD): Eliminates complicated carbohydrates and focuses on easily digested foods to reduce inflammation and support gut repair. Some people with Crohn's disease may find relief from symptoms by following the SCD, although more study is needed to prove its effectiveness.
-Elimination Diet: Involves carefully eliminating possible trigger foods from the diet and then gradually returning them to find specific food allergies or intolerances that may worsen symptoms.

-Anti-inflammatory Diet: Emphasizes whole, nutrient-dense foods that are rich in antioxidants, vitamins, minerals, and omega-3 fatty acids to lower inflammation and support general health. This diet may include fruits, veggies, fatty fish, nuts, seeds, and healthy fats while reducing processed foods, sugary sugars, and heavy fats.

Common Dietary Challenges and Solutions

Navigating food difficulties is a major part of treating Crohn's disease. Individuals with Crohn's disease often face various food hurdles that can impact symptom control, nutritional intake, and general well-being.

Here are some common food issues faced by people with Crohn's disease, along with possible solutions:

Trigger Foods: Identifying and avoiding trigger foods that worsen symptoms is a common task for people with Crohn's disease. These trigger foods can vary from person to person but may include hot foods, high-fat foods, dairy products, gluten-containing grains, and certain raw fruits and veggies. Keeping a food log and paying attention to symptom trends can help people identify their trigger foods. Once found, avoiding trigger foods and adding different choices can help reduce symptom flare-ups.

Nutritional shortages: Malabsorption of nutrients due to inflammation and damage to the gut can lead to shortages in vitamins, minerals, and other important nutrients. Common food deficits in Crohn's disease include vitamin D, vitamin B12, iron, calcium, and magnesium. Supplementing with vitamins and minerals, as suggested by a healthcare source, can help address food deficits and support general health. Additionally, eating nutrient-dense foods and focusing on a well-balanced diet can help meet nutritional goals.

High-Fiber Foods: While fiber is important for gut health, some people with Crohn's disease may have trouble handling high-fiber foods, especially during flare-ups. High-fiber foods such as raw fruits and veggies, whole grains, nuts, and seeds can worsen symptoms such as gas, bloating, and diarrhea. Opting for cooked or peeled fruits and veggies, choosing low-fiber grains such as white rice and refined pasta, and gradually increasing fiber intake can help improve tolerance to high-fiber foods.

Dietary limits: Following dietary limits, such as a low-FODMAP diet or specific carbohydrate diet (SCD), can be difficult for people with Crohn's disease. These dietary methods limit certain types of starches that can react in the gut and cause stomach complaints. Working with a registered dietitian or healthcare provider to develop a personalized nutrition plan that aligns with dietary restrictions while meeting nutritional needs can help individuals manage symptoms and achieve better symptom control.

Meal Planning and Preparation: Planning and preparing meals can be challenging for individuals with Crohn's disease, especially during flare-ups or periods of fatigue. Simplifying dinner preparation by batch cooking, meal prepping, and using comfort foods can help save time and energy. Additionally, having a well-stocked pantry and freezer with healthy staples and easy-to-prepare meal choices can make meal planning more doable.

Hydration: Chronic diarrhea and higher fluid losses linked with Crohn's disease can lead to dehydration and chemical issues. Staying hydrated by drinking plenty of fluids, including water, herbal teas, and electrolyte-rich drinks, is important for keeping hydration and supporting general health. Carrying a water bottle and setting notes to drink fluids throughout the day can help people stay hydrated.

Social Situations: Managing Crohn's disease in social situations, such as eating out with friends or visiting social events, can be difficult due to food limits and worries about symptom flare-ups. Communicating dietary needs and tastes to hosts or restaurant staff, studying menu choices in advance, and taking a snack or meal to social events can help people manage social settings while sticking to their dietary requirements.

BUILDING A CROHN'S-FRIENDLY PANTRY

Building a Crohn's-friendly kitchen is an important step in controlling Crohn's disease, a chronic inflammatory condition of the digestive tract. A well-stocked kitchen can provide people with Crohn's disease with healthy, easy-to-digest choices that support symptom control and general well-being. Here's how to build a Crohn's-friendly pantry:

Whole Grains opt for easily edible whole grains such as white rice, white pasta, sweetened bread, and oatmeal. These grains are lower in fiber and less likely to cause stomach complaints such as gas, bloating, and diarrhea compared to high-fiber oats. Choose low-fiber choices such as canned or cooked fruits and veggies without skins or seeds, canned beans, and peeling potatoes. These foods are easier on the digestive system and less likely to worsen symptoms. Include lean protein sources that are easy to digest, such as skinless chicken, fish, eggs, tofu, and canned beans. These protein choices provide important nutrients and support muscle health without causing stomach discomfort. Incorporate healthy fats such as olive oil, avocado oil, nuts, and seeds into your kitchen. These fats provide important fatty acids and support general health without worsening symptoms.
Stock up on canned foods such as canned fruits, veggies, beans, and fish. Canned choices are handy, shelf-stable, and easy to add into meals and snacks.

Nutrient-dense foods includes nutrient-dense choices such as nut butter, canned salmon or tuna, dried veggies, and shelf-stable milk replacements (such as almond milk or lactose-free milk). These foods provide important nutrients and can be easily added into a Crohn's-friendly diet. Keep refreshing liquids such as water, herbal teas, electrolyte-rich drinks, and low-acid fruit juices on hand. Staying hydrated is important for gut health and general well-being, especially for people with Crohn's disease. Use herbs, spices, and seasonings to add flavor to your food without worsening stomach problems. Common Crohn's-friendly choices include ginger, turmeric, cinnamon, and mild herbs such as parsley, basil, and dill. You can have Crohn's-friendly snack options ready, such as rice cakes, pretzels, low-fiber rackers, canned fruit in juice, and nut butter packs. These snacks provide energy and fill hunger without causing stomach pain. Consider having meal replacement choices such as protein shakes, healthy drinks, and meal replacement bars on hand for times when cooking or eating solid foods is difficult. Discuss with your healthcare provider the possible need for digestive supplements such as probiotics, digestive enzymes, and fiber supplements to support gut health and digestion.

By stocking your kitchen with Crohn's-friendly options, you can create a helpful setting that makes it easier to follow a healthy diet, control symptoms, and improve your general health and well-being. Regularly reviewing and refilling your kitchen items ensures that you always have the essentials on hand to support your dietary needs and tastes.

FOODS TO INCLUDE AND AVOID:

When treating Crohn's disease, choosing the right foods can make a significant difference in symptom control and general well-being. Here are some things to include and avoid in a Crohn's-friendly diet:

Foods to Include:
Low-Fiber Fruits and Vegetables: Opt for cooked or canned fruits and vegetables without skins or seeds, such as applesauce, mashed potatoes, carrots, and bananas. These choices are easier to digest and less likely to cause pain to the digestive system.

Lean Proteins: Choose lean protein sources such as skinless chicken, fish, eggs, tofu, and well-cooked soft meats. These choices provide important nutrients without adding extra fat or fiber.

Low-Fiber Grains: Select easily digestible grains such as white rice, white pasta, sweetened bread, and oatmeal. These choices are lower in fiber and less likely to cause stomach pain.

Healthy Fats: Incorporate healthy fats such as olive oil, avocado oil, nuts, and seeds into your diet. These fats provide important fatty acids and support general health without worsening symptoms.

Lactose-Free or Low-Lactose Dairy: Choose lactose-free or low-lactose dairy choices such as lactose-free milk, yogurt, and hard cheeses. These options are easier to digest and less likely to cause stomach complaints in people with lactose intolerance.

Hydrating Beverages: Stay hydrated with water, herbal teas, electrolyte-rich drinks, and low-acid fruit juices. Proper water is important for gut health and general well-being.

Probiotic Foods: Incorporate probiotic-rich foods such as yogurt, kefir, cabbage, and kimchi into your diet. Probiotics can help promote a healthy mix of gut bacteria and support stomach health.

Soft or Pureed Foods: During flare-ups or times of stomach pain, opt for softer or pureed foods that are easier to handle, such as soups, shakes, and pureed veggies.

Foods to Avoid:

High-Fiber Foods: Limit or avoid high-fiber foods such as raw fruits and veggies, whole grains, nuts, seeds, and tough cuts of meat. These foods can be tough to digest and may worsen symptoms.

Spicy Foods: Avoid spicy foods, hot sauces, and peppers, as they can upset the digestive system and cause symptoms such as stomach pain and diarrhea.

High-Fat Foods: Limit or avoid high-fat foods such as fried foods, fatty cuts of meat, thick sauces, and rich sweets. These foods can exacerbate symptoms and may add to stomach pain.

Dairy Products (if Lactose Intolerant): If you are lactose intolerant, limit or avoid dairy products such as milk, cheese, and ice cream, as they can cause stomach symptoms such as gas, bloating, and diarrhea.

caffeine and fizzy Beverages: Limit or avoid caffeine beverages such as coffee, tea, and pop, as well as fizzy drinks, as they can upset the stomach system and increase symptoms.

Alcohol and Sugary drinks: Limit or avoid alcohol drinks, as they can add to stomach discomfort and may worsen symptoms. Avoid high-sugar and processed foods such as candy, sweets, sugary cereals, and processed snacks, as they can add to inflammation and stomach pain.

Artificial Sweeteners: Limit or avoid artificial sweeteners such as sorbitol, mannitol, and xylitol, as they can cause stomach complaints such as gas, bloating, and diarrhea in some people.

By including Crohn's-friendly foods and avoiding possible causes, people can better control their symptoms, support gut health, and improve their general quality of life. It's important to listen to your body and work with a healthcare provider or certified dietitian to build a personalized diet plan that meets your individual wants and tastes.

TIPS FOR MEAL PLANNING AND GROCERY SHOPPING:

Meal planning and grocery shopping can be difficult jobs for people handling Crohn's disease, but with some smart tips, you can make the process easier and more doable. Here are some tips for meal planning and food shopping with Crohn's disease:

Meal Planning:
Keep meal plans simple and focus on easy-to-digest, Crohn's-friendly foods. Choose recipes that require minimal preparation and include items that are gentle on the digestive system.

Consider dietary restrictions or food intolerances you may have, such as lactose intolerance or sensitivity to certain food groups. Modify recipes or replace items as needed to suit your food needs. Include variety in your meals to ensure you're getting a wide range of nutrients. Incorporate different protein sources, grains, fruits, and veggies to keep meals interesting and properly balanced. Also consider batch cooking meals in advance and portioning them out for easy grab-and-go options throughout the week. Soups, stews, casseroles, and grain bowls are all excellent choices for batch cooking.

Freeze Meals: Freeze extra parts or batch-cooked meals in individual portions for future use. Having frozen meals on hand can be useful for days when you don't feel up to cooking or need a quick meal choice.

Listen to Your Body: Pay attention to how different foods affect your symptoms and change your meal plans accordingly. If certain foods regularly cause symptoms, try ignoring or limiting them in your meal plans.

Grocery Shopping:
Make a detailed shopping list based on your meal plan to ensure you have all the items you need for the week. Organize your list by groups (e.g., fruit, dairy, cupboard items) to simplify your shopping trip, focus on shopping the edges of the grocery store, where you'll find fresh vegetables, lean meats, dairy, and other

whole foods. Limit your time in the middle lanes, which often contain prepared and packed foods.

Read Labels Carefully: When buying prepared foods, read labels carefully to check for extra sugars, fake ingredients, and other possible triggers. Choose goods with minimal ingredients and avoid those having fillers or chemicals. Keep your kitchen stocked with Crohn's-friendly staples such as low-fiber foods, canned fruits and veggies, lean meats, healthy fats, and digestive-friendly snacks. Having these things on hand makes food preparation easy.

Choose Fresh and Frozen Options: Opt for fresh or frozen fruits and vegetables over canned varieties whenever possible. Fresh fruit is nutrient-rich and can be easier to digest, while frozen choices are handy and have a longer shelf life.

Consider Convenience Foods: Don't hesitate to include convenience foods such as pre-cut fruits and veggies, pre-cooked grains, and canned beans in your buying list. These things can save time and energy during meal preparation.

Shop During Off-Peak Hours: Avoid busy food shops by shopping during off-peak hours, such as early mornings or weekdays. This can help lower worry and make your buying experience more pleasant. Remember to stay refreshed while food shopping by taking a water bottle with you and sipping water throughout your trip. Proper water is important for gut health and general well-being.

STRESS MANAGEMENT TECHNIQUES

Managing stress is important for people with Crohn's disease, as stress can worsen symptoms and negatively impact general well-being. Here are some stress control methods that can help people with Crohn's disease:

Deep Breathing: Practice deep breathing techniques to promote calm and lower stress. Sit or lie down in a comfortable position, close your eyes, and take slow, deep breaths, focused on filling your belly with air. Hold each breath for a few seconds before releasing slowly. Repeat this process for several minutes to calm your thoughts and body.

Mindfulness Meditation: Engage in mindfulness meditation to develop present-moment focus and lower stress. Find a quiet place where you won't be bothered, sit easily, and focus your mind on your breath or a specific item. Notice any thoughts, feelings, or sensations that come without judgment, and gently guide your focus back to the present moment whenever your mind wanders.

Progressive Muscle Relaxation: Practice progressive muscle relaxation to release stress and promote calm throughout your body. Start by tensing and then releasing each muscle group, starting from your toes and making your way up to your head.

Focus on the feelings of tightness and release in each muscle group, allowing yourself to let go of worry and strain with each breath.

Exercise Regularly: Engage in regular physical movement to lower stress and improve general well-being. Choose things that you enjoy, such as walks, swimming, yoga, or tai chi, and aim for at least 30 minutes of mild exercise most days of the week. Exercise releases endorphins, which are natural mood lifters that can help relieve stress and improve mood.

Maintain a Healthy Lifestyle: Prioritize self-care tasks that support physical and mental well-being, such as getting adequate sleep, eating a balanced diet, staying hydrated, and avoiding excessive alcohol and coffee. Taking care of your body and mind can help you better cope with stress and handle your Crohn's disease effectively.Seek Support: Reach out to friends, family members, or support groups for mental support and guidance. Sharing your experiences with others who understand what you're going through can help you feel less isolated and more supported in controlling your condition.

Practice Time Management: Manage your time successfully to reduce worry and overload. Break tasks down into smaller, doable steps, organize your responsibilities, and share tasks when possible. Set realistic goals and dates for yourself, and be open in changing your plans as needed.Limit Exposure to **Stressful Situations**: Identify and lessen causes of stress in your life, whether they're connected to work, relationships, or other areas of your life. Set limits to protect your time and energy, and avoid scenarios or people that cause worry whenever possible.

Engage in Relaxing Activities: Make time for activities that help you relax and unwind, such as reading, listening to music, spending time in nature, or practicing skills and interests. Doing things that bring you joy and relaxation can help lower stress and improve your general quality of life.Consider.

Professional Help: If you're fighting to handle stress on your own, consider getting help from a mental health professional such as a therapist or psychologist. They can provide you with additional coping techniques, help, and advice suited to your unique needs.

EXERCISE AND PHYSICAL ACTIVITY RECOMMENDATIONS

Exercise and physical exercise play an important part in controlling Crohn's disease by boosting general health, lowering inflammation, and improving mood and energy levels. Here are some fitness and physical movement suggestions for people with Crohn's disease:

Check Your Healthcare Provider: Before starting any exercise program, check with your healthcare provider to ensure that it's safe and appropriate for your individual situation. They can provide advice on the types and levels of exercise that are good for you.

Start Slowly: If you're new to exercise or have been idle for a while, start slowly and gradually increase the volume and length of your workouts. Begin with low-impact activities such as walking, swimming, or riding, and gradually add more difficult routines as your fitness level improves.

Choose Low-Impact Activities: Opt for low-impact activities that are gentle on the joints and digestive system, especially if you experience stomach pain or soreness. Swimming, riding, yoga, tai chi, and walking are all excellent choices for people with Crohn's disease.

Focus on Flexibility and Strength: Incorporate flexibility and strength training techniques into your practice to improve movement, stability, and muscle power. Pilates, yoga, and manual movements such as squats, lunges, and dips can help strengthen the core muscles and improve general health.

Listen to Your Body: Pay attention to how your body reacts to exercise and change your schedule accordingly. If you feel pain, tiredness, or other signs during or after activity, take a break and rest. It's important to listen to your body's cues and not push yourself too hard.

Stay Hydrated: Drink plenty of water before, during, and after exercise to stay hydrated and support digestion. Dehydration can exacerbate symptoms and increase the risk of problems, so it's important to drink enough fluids, especially during hard workouts or in hot weather.

Manage Stress: Use exercise as a tool to manage stress and improve happiness. Engaging in regular physical exercise can help lower worry, anxiety, and sadness, which are typical signs of Crohn's disease. Find things that you enjoy and that help you relax and unwind.

Be Consistent: Aim for stability in your exercise practice by booking regular workouts throughout the week. Even small bouts of exercise can have benefits, so try to add physical movement into your daily routine whenever possible.

Warm Up and Cool Down: Always warm up before exercise and cool down later to avoid harm and ease muscle soreness. Spend a few minutes doing active stretches or light jogging before your workout, and finish with motionless stretches to improve flexibility and promote rest.

Consider Professional Guidance: If you're unsure about how to safely and effectively exercise with Crohn's disease, consider working with a trained fitness trainer or physical therapist who has experience working with people with chronic illnesses. They can provide personalized advice and support to help you meet your exercise goals while controlling your condition effectively.

NOURISHING RECIPES FOR WELLNESS

Nourishing recipes play a vital role in supporting overall wellness, especially for individuals managing Crohn's disease. Every meal is an opportunity for triumph—a chance to fuel your body with healing, comforting, and nourishing foods. Each dish is carefully crafted not only to tantalize your taste buds but to nurture your body. From comforting soups that soothe inflamed bellies to vibrant salads bursting with nutrients, every bite is a step towards reclaiming your vitality and embracing wellness. It's about taking back control of your health, finding joy in the kitchen, and discovering the transformative power of food. It's a reminder that even in the midst of hardship, there is beauty, there is healing, and there is hope.

Here are some nourishing recipe ideas that are gentle on the digestive system and packed with essential nutrients to support health and well-being:

BREAKFAST

BANANA OATMEAL BREAKFAST BOWL

PREP TIME: 15 MIN COOK TIME: 10 MIN TOTAL TIME: 25 MIN

SERVINGS: 1

NUTRITIONAL INFORMATION (PER SERVING)

CAL: 250K PROTEIN: 6G CARB: 30G FAT: 3G FIBER: 6G SUGAR: 5G

INGREDIENTS

1/2 cup rolled oats

1 cup water or milk of your choice

1 ripe banana, mashed

Optional toppings: Sliced banana, nuts, honey or maple syrup

DIRECTIONS

Bring milk or water to a boil in a small pot. Turn down the heat and add the rolled oats. Cook for 5 to 10 minutes, stirring every now and then, until the consistency you want is reached. Mix in the mashed banana until everything is well mixed. Take it off the heat, put it in a bowl, and add any toppings you want.

<u>SCRAMBLED EGGS WITH SPINACH</u>

PREP TIME: 15 MIN COOK TIME: 10 MIN TOTAL TIME: 25 MIN

SERVINGS: 1

NUTRITIONAL INFORMATION (PER SERVING)

CAL: 300K   PROTEIN: 15G   CARB: 5G   FAT: 20G   FIBER: 1G   SUGAR: 1G

<u>INGREDIENTS</u>

2 eggs

1 cup fresh spinach leaves

Salt and pepper to taste

Olive oil or cooking spray

<u>DIRECTIONS</u>

Add the eggs, salt, and pepper to a bowl and whisk them together. Put the pan on medium heat and spray it with cooking spray or olive oil. Put spinach in the pan and cook for about two minutes, until it wilts. Add eggs to the spinach and beat them for three to four minutes, or until they are fully cooked. Warm up and serve.

GREEK YOGURT PARFAIT

PREP TIME: 15 MIN COOK TIME: MIN TOTAL TIME: 15 MIN

SERVINGS: 1

NUTRITIONAL INFORMATION (PER SERVING)
CAL: 300K PROTEIN: 20G CARB: 30G FAT: 8G FIBER: 6G SUGAR: 15G

INGREDIENTS

1 cup Greek yogurt
1/2 cup granola
1/2 cup mixed berries (such as strawberries, blueberries, raspberries)

DIRECTIONS

In a glass or dish, combine the Greek yogurt, granola, and mixed berries.
Repeat layering until the ingredients are well mixed.
Serve immediately.

QUINOA BREAKFAST BOWL

PREP TIME: 15 MIN COOK TIME: MIN TOTAL TIME: 15 MIN
SERVINGS: 1
NUTRITIONAL INFORMATION (PER SERVING)
CAL: 300K PROTEIN: 7G CARB: 20G FAT: 6G FIBER: 3G SUGAR: 20G

INGREDIENTS

1/2 cup cooked quinoa
1/2 cup almond milk
1 tablespoon honey or maple syrup
1/4 teaspoon ground cinnamon
Sliced bananas, nuts, and dried fruits for topping

DIRECTIONS

In a bowl, combine cooked quinoa, almond milk, honey or maple syrup, and
cinnamon.
Top with sliced bananas, almonds, and dried fruit.
Serve either warm or cooled.

OATMEAL WITH APPLESAUCE, CINNAMON, AND SOY YOGURT.

PREP TIME: 5 MIN COOK TIME: 15 MIN TOTAL TIME: 20 MIN
SERVINGS: 1
NUTRITIONAL INFORMATION (PER SERVING)
CAL: 250K PROTEIN: 8G CARB: 30G FAT: 6G FIBER: 7G SUGAR: 10G

INGREDIENTS

1 cup old-fashioned oats
2 cups milk (dairy or nondairy - I used unsweetened almond milk)
2 tablespoons ground flaxseed
1 apple, cut into small cubes
2 tablespoons honey
1 teaspoon ground cinnamon

DIRECTIONS

Combine all of the oatmeal ingredients in a medium pot. Bring the mixture to a boil over medium-high heat, then reduce to a simmer for 10-12 minutes, or until the oatmeal thickens and the apples are slightly softened.

For the sauteed apple topping: Melt the butter in a nonstick pan over medium heat. Add the chopped apples and simmer for 2-3 minutes, stirring periodically, until they soften. Reduce the heat to low, then add the honey and cinnamon. Stir and heat for a further 2-3 minutes, or until the apples are just soft and the honey bubbles.

Divide the oats into two dishes and top with sautéed apples, yogurt, and walnuts.

<u>RICE CAKE WITH PEANUT BUTTER</u>

PREP TIME: 15 MIN COOK TIME: MIN TOTAL TIME: 15MIN
SERVINGS: 1
NUTRITIONAL INFORMATION (PER SERVING)
CAL: 200K PROTEIN: 5G CARB: 15G FAT: 12G FIBER: 3G SUGAR: 5G

INGREDIENTS

1 rice cake
2 tablespoons peanut butter
Sliced banana or berries for topping

DIRECTIONS

Spread peanut butter evenly on top of the rice cake.
Top with sliced banana or berries.
Serve immediately.

SAUTÉED VEGETABLE OMELETTE

PREP TIME: 15 MIN COOK TIME: MIN TOTAL TIME: 15MIN

SERVINGS: 1

NUTRITIONAL INFORMATION (PER SERVING)
CAL: 200K PROTEIN: 14G CARB: 5G FAT: 12G FIBER: 2G SUGAR: 2G

INGREDIENTS

2 eggs
1/4 cup diced bell peppers
1/4 cup diced onions
1/4 cup diced tomatoes
Handful of spinach
Salt and pepper to taste
Cooking spray or olive oil

DIRECTIONS

In a mixing dish, combine eggs, salt, and pepper.

Coat a skillet with cooking spray or olive oil.

Add the bell peppers, onions, and tomatoes to the skillet. Sauté for 2-3 minutes, until softened.

Cook the spinach in the pan until it has wilted.

Pour the beaten eggs over the veggies and simmer until set, approximately 3-4 minutes.

Fold the omelet in half and place on a platter.

Serve hot.

<u>COTTAGE CHEESE AND FRUIT</u>

PREP TIME: 15 MIN COOK TIME: MIN TOTAL TIME: 15MIN

SERVINGS: 1

NUTRITIONAL INFORMATION (PER SERVING)

CAL: 150K PROTEIN: 5G CARB: 15G FAT: 3G FIBER: 4G SUGAR: 10G

<u>INGREDIENTS</u>

1/2 cup low-fat cottage cheese

1/2 cup mixed berries (such as strawberries, blueberries, raspberries)

Optional toppings: Nuts, seeds, honey or maple syrup

<u>DIRECTIONS</u>

In a bowl, serve cottage cheese topped with mixed berries.

Add optional toppings if desired.

Serve immediately.

OVERNIGHT OATS

PREP TIME: 15 MIN COOK TIME: MIN TOTAL TIME: 4+ hours (overnight)

SERVINGS: 1

NUTRITIONAL INFORMATION (PER SERVING)
CAL: 300K PROTEIN: 8G CARB: 25G FAT: 10G FIBER: 8G SUGAR: 10G

INGREDIENTS

1/2 cup rolled oats
1/2 cup almond milk
1 tablespoon chia seeds
1 tablespoon honey or maple syrup
Sliced fruits, nuts, seeds for topping

DIRECTIONS

In a jar or dish, combine the rolled oats, almond milk, chia seeds, and honey or maple syrup.
Cover and refrigerate overnight, or at least 4 hours.
Stir thoroughly before serving and garnish with cut fruits, nuts, and seeds.

<u>SWEET POTATO HASH</u>

PREP TIME: 15 MIN COOK TIME: 15MIN TOTAL TIME: 30MIN

SERVINGS: 1

NUTRITIONAL INFORMATION (PER SERVING)

CAL: 200K **PROTEIN:** 3G **CARB:** 25G **FAT:** 2G **FIBER:** 6G **SUGAR:** 10G

INGREDIENTS

1 medium sweet potato, peeled and diced

1/4 cup diced bell peppers

1/4 cup diced onions

1/4 teaspoon paprika

Salt and pepper to taste

Cooking spray or olive oil

DIRECTIONS

Coat a skillet with cooking spray or olive oil over medium heat.

Cook sweet potatoes in the skillet for 5-10 minutes, until tender.

Add the bell peppers, onions, paprika, salt, and pepper to the skillet. Cook for a further 3-5 minutes, until the veggies are soft.

Serve hot.

COCONUT YOGURT WITH ALMONDS

PREP TIME: 15 MIN COOK TIME: 15MIN TOTAL TIME: 30MIN

SERVINGS: 1

NUTRITIONAL INFORMATION (PER SERVING)

CAL: 200K PROTEIN: 10G CARB: 10G FAT: 12G FIBER: 3G SUGAR: 5G

INGREDIENTS

1/2 cup coconut yogurt

2 tablespoons sliced almonds

Sliced fruits for topping

DIRECTIONS

In a bowl, serve coconut yogurt topped with sliced almonds.

Add sliced fruits on top.

Serve immediately.

RICE PORRIDGE

PREP TIME: 15 MIN COOK TIME: 15MIN TOTAL TIME: 30MIN

SERVINGS: 1

NUTRITIONAL INFORMATION (PER SERVING)
CAL: 250K PROTEIN: 5G CARB: 28G FAT: 4G FIBER: 3G SUGAR: 15G

INGREDIENTS

1/2 cup cooked rice

1 cup almond milk

1 tablespoon honey or maple syrup

1/4 teaspoon ground cinnamon

Sliced fruits, nuts, and seeds for topping

DIRECTIONS

In a saucepan, mix the cooked rice, almond milk, honey or maple syrup, and ground cinnamon.
Bring to a simmer over medium heat, then boil for 5-7 minutes, stirring periodically, until thick.
Serve warm, topped with sliced fruits, nuts, and seeds.

AVOCADO TOAST

PREP TIME: 15 MIN COOK TIME: 15MIN TOTAL TIME: 30MIN

SERVINGS: 1

NUTRITIONAL INFORMATION (PER SERVING)
CAL: 200K PROTEIN: 4G CARB: 20G FAT: 12G FIBER: 8G SUGAR: 2G

INGREDIENTS

1 slice whole grain bread, toasted

1/2 ripe avocado, mashed

Salt and pepper to taste

Optional toppings: Sliced tomatoes, red pepper flakes, hemp seeds

DIRECTIONS

Spread mashed avocado evenly on top of the toasted bread.

Season with salt and pepper to taste.

Add optional toppings if desired.

Serve immediately.

FRITTATA MUFFINS

PREP TIME: 15 MIN COOK TIME: 15MIN TOTAL TIME: 30MIN

SERVINGS: 1

NUTRITIONAL INFORMATION (PER SERVING)

CAL: 70K PROTEIN: 5G CARB: 2G FAT: 4G FIBER: 1G SUGAR: 1G

INGREDIENTS

6 large eggs
1/4 cup milk (dairy or dairy-free)
1/2 cup chopped spinach
1/4 cup diced bell pepper
1/4 cup diced onion
1/4 cup diced tomatoes
1/4 cup shredded cheddar cheese (optional)
Salt and pepper to taste
Cooking spray or olive oil for greasing muffin tin

DIRECTIONS

Preheat the oven to 350°F (175° C). Coat a muffin tray with cooking spray or olive oil. In a mixing dish, break the eggs and whisk in the milk until well blended. Mix in the chopped spinach, diced bell pepper, onion, and tomatoes. If desired, add some shredded cheddar cheese.

Season the mixture with salt and pepper to taste, then whisk until all of the ingredients are uniformly dispersed.

Pour the egg mixture into the muffin cups, filling them approximately 3/4 full. Bake in a preheated oven for 20-25 minutes, or until the tops are firm and faintly brown. Remove the muffin tray from the oven and allow the frittata muffins to cool for a few minutes before gently removing them.

Serve warm or room temperature. Enjoy!

LUNCH RECIPE

QUINOA SALAD WITH GRILLED CHICKEN

PREP TIME: 15 MIN COOK TIME: 20 MIN (for quinoa) TOTAL TIME: 35

MIN

SERVINGS: 2

NUTRITIONAL INFORMATION (PER SERVING)

CAL: 300K   PROTEIN: 25G   CARB: 20G   FAT: 15G   FIBER: 5G   SUGAR: 5G

INGREDIENTS

1 cup cooked quinoa

1 grilled chicken breast, sliced

Mixed salad greens

Cherry tomatoes, halved

Cucumber, diced

Red onion, thinly sliced

Feta cheese, crumbled

Balsamic vinaigrette dressing

DIRECTIONS:

In a large bowl, combine cooked quinoa, grilled chicken slices, mixed salad greens, cherry tomatoes, cucumber, red onion, and feta cheese.

Drizzle with balsamic vinaigrette dressing and toss to combine.

Serve chilled.

TURKEY AND AVOCADO WRAP

PREP TIME: 15 MIN COOK TIME: 20 MIN (for quinoa) TOTAL TIME: 35

MIN

SERVINGS: 2

NUTRITIONAL INFORMATION (PER SERVING)

CAL: 350K PROTEIN: 30G   CARB: 25G FAT: 20G FIBER: 8G SUGAR: 3G

INGREDIENTS

2 whole grain wraps

8 ounces sliced turkey breast

1 avocado, sliced

Mixed salad greens

Sliced tomatoes

Dijon mustard

Optional: Sprouts, shredded carrots

DIRECTIONS:

Lay out the whole grain wraps on a flat surface.

Divide the sliced turkey breast, avocado slices, mixed salad greens, and sliced tomatoes evenly between the wraps.

Drizzle with Dijon mustard.

Optional: Add sprouts and shredded carrots.

Roll up the wraps tightly and slice in half.

Serve immediately.

SALMON AND VEGETABLE STIR-FRY

PREP TIME: 15 MIN COOK TIME: 15MIN TOTAL TIME: 30MIN

SERVINGS: 2

NUTRITIONAL INFORMATION (PER SERVING, WITHOUT RICE/QUINOA)

CAL: 250K PROTEIN: 20G CARB: 15G FAT: 12G FIBER: 5G SUGAR: 5G

INGREDIENTS

8 ounces salmon fillet, cut into cubes

2 cups mixed vegetables (bell peppers, broccoli, carrots)

2 cloves garlic, minced

1 tablespoon soy sauce

1 tablespoon hoisin sauce

1 tablespoon sesame oil

Cooked brown rice or quinoa for serving

DIRECTIONS

Heat the sesame oil in a large pan over medium heat.

Sauté the minced garlic for 1 minute.

Cook the salmon cubes until browned on both sides, approximately 3-4 minutes.

Cook the mixed veggies in the skillet for approximately 5 minutes, or until soft and crisp.

Cook a further 2 minutes after adding the soy sauce and hoisin sauce.

Serve the fish and vegetable stir fry with cooked brown rice or quinoa.

VEGETABLE AND LENTIL SOUP

PREP TIME: 25 MIN COOK TIME: 15MIN TOTAL TIME: 40MIN

SERVINGS: 4

NUTRITIONAL INFORMATION (PER SERVING)

CAL: 200K PROTEIN: 12G CARB: 25G FAT: 1G FIBER: 10G SUGAR: 15G

INGREDIENTS

1 cup cooked lentils

4 cups vegetable broth

2 cups mixed vegetables (carrots, celery, onions)

2 cloves garlic, minced

1 teaspoon dried thyme

Salt and pepper to taste

Fresh parsley for garnish

DIRECTIONS

In a large saucepan, boil the vegetable broth over medium heat.

Add the mixed veggies, minced garlic, dry thyme, salt, and pepper to the saucepan.

Simmer for 15-20 minutes, until the veggies are soft.

Stir in the cooked lentils and heat for a further 5 minutes.

Taste and adjust the seasoning as required.

Serve hot and garnished with fresh parsley.

QUINOA STUFFED BELL PEPPERS

PREP TIME: 15 MIN COOK TIME: 35MIN TOTAL TIME: 50MIN

SERVINGS: 3

NUTRITIONAL INFORMATION (PER SERVING)
CAL: 300K PROTEIN: 15G CARB: 10G FAT: 5G FIBER: 12G SUGAR: 8G

INGREDIENTS

4 bell peppers, halved and seeds removed
1 cup cooked quinoa
1 cup black beans, drained and rinsed
1 cup corn kernels
1 cup diced tomatoes
1 teaspoon chili powder
1/2 teaspoon cumin
Salt and pepper to taste
Optional: Shredded cheese, avocado slices, salsa for topping

DIRECTIONS

Preheat the oven to 375° Fahrenheit (190° Celsius). Place the bell pepper halves in a baking dish.

In a large mixing bowl, combine cooked quinoa, black beans, corn kernels, chopped tomatoes, chili powder, cumin, salt, and pepper.

Spoon the quinoa mixture into each bell pepper half.

Cover the baking dish with foil and bake for 25-30 minutes, until the peppers are cooked.

Remove the foil, sprinkle with shredded cheese (if using), and bake for another 5 minutes, or until the cheese has melted.

Serve the filled bell peppers hot, topped with avocado slices and salsa if preferred.

CHICKEN AND VEGETABLE SKEWER

PREP TIME: 15 MIN COOK TIME: 15MIN TOTAL TIME: 30MIN

SERVINGS: 2

NUTRITIONAL INFORMATION (PER SERVING)

CAL: 250K PROTEIN: 25G CARB: 5G FAT: 12G FIBER: 5G SUGAR: 5G

INGREDIENTS

8 ounces chicken breast, cut into cubes
2 cups mixed vegetables (such as bell peppers, zucchini, onions)
2 tablespoons olive oil
1 teaspoon dried Italian herbs (basil, oregano, thyme)
Salt and pepper to taste

DIRECTIONS

Preheat the grill or grill pan to medium-high heat.

In a mixing dish, combine the chicken cubes and mixed veggies with the olive oil, dried Italian herbs, salt, and pepper.

Thread chicken and veggies alternately onto skewers.

Grill the skewers for 10-12 minutes, flipping regularly, until the chicken is fully cooked and the veggies are soft.

Serve hot.

SPINACH AND FETA TURKEY BURGERS

PREP TIME: 15 MIN COOK TIME: 15MIN TOTAL TIME: 30MIN

SERVINGS: 2

NUTRITIONAL INFORMATION (PER SERVING)

CAL: 200K PROTEIN: 20G CARB: 5G FAT: 10G FIBER: 2G SUGAR: 1G

INGREDIENTS

8 ounces ground turkey

1 cup fresh spinach, chopped

1/4 cup crumbled feta cheese

1/4 cup breadcrumbs

1 egg

2 cloves garlic, minced

Salt and pepper to taste

Whole grain burger buns

Lettuce, tomato slices, red onion slices for topping

DIRECTIONS

In a large bowl, combine ground turkey, chopped spinach, crumbled feta cheese, breadcrumbs, egg, minced garlic, salt, and pepper.

Mix until well combined, then form into burger patties.

Heat a grill or skillet over medium heat. Cook the turkey burgers for about 5-6 minutes per side, or until cooked through.

Toast the whole grain burger buns if desired.

Serve turkey burgers on buns with lettuce, tomato slices, and red onion slices.

GREEK SALAD WITH GRILLED SHRIMP

PREP TIME: 15 MIN COOK TIME: 10MIN TOTAL TIME: 25MIN

SERVINGS: 2

NUTRITIONAL INFORMATION (PER SERVING)
CAL: 250K PROTEIN: 25G CARB: 10G FAT: 10G FIBER: 5G SUGAR: 5G

INGREDIENTS

8 ounces shrimp, peeled and deveined
4 cups mixed salad greens
Cherry tomatoes, halved
Cucumber, diced
Red onion, thinly sliced
Kalamata olives
Feta cheese, crumbled
Greek vinaigrette dressing

DIRECTIONS

Preheat grill or grill pan over medium-high heat.

Season shrimp with salt and pepper, then grill for 2-3 minutes per side until pink and cooked through.

In a big bowl, blend mixed salad leaves, cherry tomatoes, cucumber, red onion, Kalamata olives, and feta cheese.

Add cooked shrimp on top.

Drizzle with Greek vinegar sauce and toss to mix.

Serve quickly.

ZUCCHINI NOODLES WITH PESTO

PREP TIME: 15 MIN COOK TIME: 10MIN TOTAL TIME: 25MIN

SERVINGS: 2

NUTRITIONAL INFORMATION (PER SERVING)

CAL: 200K PROTEIN: 5G CARB: 10G FAT: 15G FIBER: 5G SUGAR: 5G

INGREDIENTS

2 medium zucchini, spiralized

1/4 cup homemade or store-bought pesto

Cherry tomatoes, halved

Pine nuts, toasted

Fresh basil leaves for garnish

Optional: Grated Parmesan cheese

DIRECTIONS

Heat a pan over medium heat. Add spiralized zucchini noodles and cook for 2-3 minutes until slightly softer.

Transfer zucchini noodles to a bowl and toss with pesto until well coated.

Divide zucchini noodles into serving bowls.

Top with cherry tomatoes, toasted pine nuts, fresh basil leaves, and grated Parmesan cheese if preferred.

Serve quickly.

TUNA SALAD LETTUCE WRAPS

PREP TIME: 15 MIN COOK TIME: 10MIN TOTAL TIME: 25MIN

SERVINGS: 2

NUTRITIONAL INFORMATION (PER SERVING)

CAL: 150K PROTEIN: 25G CARB: 5G FAT: 5G FIBER: 2G SUGAR: 3G

INGREDIENTS

1 can (5 ounces) tuna, drained

1/4 cup diced celery

1/4 cup diced red onion

1/4 cup diced pickles

2 tablespoons Greek yogurt or mayonnaise

1 teaspoon Dijon mustard

Salt and pepper to taste

Lettuce leaves for wrapping

DIRECTIONS

In a basin, combine together tuna, diced celery, diced red onion, diced pickles, Greek yogurt or mayonnaise, Dijon mustard, salt, and pepper.

Spoon tuna salad onto lettuce leaves.

Roll up the lettuce leaves to form bundles.

Serve immediately.

<u>VEGETABLE AND QUINOA STUFFED PORTOBELLO MUSHROOMS</u>

PREP TIME: 25 MIN COOK TIME: 20MIN TOTAL TIME: 45MIN

SERVINGS: 4

NUTRITIONAL INFORMATION (PER SERVING)

CAL: 200K PROTEIN: 10G CARB: 10G FAT: 5G FIBER: 6G SUGAR: 4G

INGREDIENTS

4 large Portobello mushrooms

1 cup cooked quinoa

1 cup mixed vegetables (such as bell peppers, onions, zucchini)

2 cloves garlic, minced

1/4 cup grated Parmesan cheese

Salt and pepper to taste

Olive oil for drizzling

DIRECTIONS

Preheat oven to 375°F (190°C). Remove stems from Portobello mushrooms and delicately scoop out the gills.

In a basin, combine together cooked quinoa, assorted vegetables, minced garlic, grated Parmesan cheese, salt, and pepper.

Stuff each Portobello mushroom with the quinoa mixture.

Drizzle with olive oil and set on a baking sheet.

Bake for 20-25 minutes until mushrooms are tender and filling is heated through

Serve heated.

<u>SHRIMP AND AVOCADO SALAD</u>

PREP TIME: 25 MIN COOK TIME: 20MIN TOTAL TIME: 45MIN

SERVINGS: 4

NUTRITIONAL INFORMATION (PER SERVING)

CAL: 250K PROTEIN: 25G CARB: 15G FAT: 10G FIBER: 8G SUGAR: 5G

INGREDIENTS

8 ounces shrimp, peeled and deveined

4 cups mixed salad greens

Cherry tomatoes, halved

Cucumber, diced

Avocado, diced

Red onion, thinly sliced

Lemon vinaigrette dressing

DIRECTIONS

Heat a skillet over medium-high heat. Add shrimp and sauté for 2-3 minutes per side until pink and heated through.

In a large basin, incorporate assorted salad greens, cherry tomatoes, cucumber, avocado, and red onion.

Add fried prawns on top.

Drizzle with lemon vinaigrette dressing and whisk to combine.

Serve immediately.

<u>EGGPLANT AND CHICKPEA CURRY</u>

PREP TIME: 15 MIN COOK TIME: 25MIN TOTAL TIME: 40MIN

SERVINGS: 4

NUTRITIONAL INFORMATION (PER SERVING)

CAL: 250K PROTEIN: 10G CARB: 11G FAT: 5G FIBER: 12G SUGAR: 10G

INGREDIENTS

1 large eggplant, diced

1 can (15 ounces) chickpeas, drained and rinsed

1 can (14 ounces) diced tomatoes

1 onion, chopped

2 cloves garlic, minced

1 tablespoon curry powder

1 teaspoon ground cumin

1/2 teaspoon ground coriander

1/4 teaspoon cayenne pepper (optional)

Salt and pepper to taste

Fresh cilantro for garnish

Cooked brown rice for serving

DIRECTIONS

In a large skillet, heat olive oil over medium heat. Sauté the chopped onion and minced garlic for 2-3 minutes, until softened.

Cook the diced eggplant in the pan for 5-7 minutes, or until gently browned.

Mix in the chickpeas, chopped tomatoes, curry powder, ground cumin, ground coriander, cayenne pepper (if using), salt, and pepper.

Cover and cook for 15-20 minutes, stirring periodically, until the eggplant is cooked.

Taste and adjust the seasoning as required.

Serve eggplant and chickpea stew hot, topped with fresh cilantro and cooked brown rice.

MEDITERRANEAN VEGGIE WRAP

PREP TIME: 15 MIN COOK TIME: 15MIN TOTAL TIME: 30MIN

SERVINGS: 4

NUTRITIONAL INFORMATION (PER SERVING)
CAL: 300K PROTEIN: 10G CARB: 19G FAT: 15G FIBER: 8G SUGAR: 5G

INGREDIENTS

2 whole grain wraps
1/2 cup hummus
1/2 cup mixed salad greens
Cherry tomatoes, halved
Cucumber, thinly sliced
Red onion, thinly sliced
Kalamata olives, sliced
Feta cheese, crumbled
Fresh parsley for garnish

DIRECTIONS

Spread out the whole grain wrappers on a level surface.

Spread the hummus evenly on the wrappers.

Add mixed salad greens, cherry tomatoes, cucumber, red onion, Kalamata olives, and crumbled feta cheese on top.

Sprinkle with fresh parsley.

Roll the wraps securely and cut in half.

Serve immediately.

TOFU STIR-FRY WITH BROWN RICE

PREP TIME: 15 MIN COOK TIME: 15MIN TOTAL TIME: 30MIN

SERVINGS: 4

NUTRITIONAL INFORMATION (PER SERVING)
CAL: 250K PROTEIN: 15G CARB: 15G FAT: 12G FIBER: 5G SUGAR: 5G

INGREDIENTS

8 ounces extra-firm tofu, pressed and cubed
2 cups mixed vegetables (such as bell peppers, broccoli, snap peas)
2 cloves garlic, minced
1 tablespoon soy sauce
1 tablespoon hoisin sauce
1 tablespoon sesame oil
Cooked brown rice for serving

DIRECTIONS

Heat the sesame oil in a large pan or wok over medium heat.

Sauté the minced garlic for 1 minute.

Cook the cubed tofu in the pan until browned on both sides, which should take around 5-7 minutes.

Stir-fry the mixed veggies in the pan for a further 5 minutes, or until tender and crisp.

Cook a further 2 minutes after adding the soy sauce and hoisin sauce.

Serve the tofu stir-fry over cooked brown rice.

DINNER RECIPE

BAKED SALMON WITH ROASTED VEGETABLES

PREP TIME: 15 MIN COOK TIME: 20MIN TOTAL TIME: 35MIN

SERVINGS: 3

NUTRITIONAL INFORMATION (PER SERVING)

CAL: 250K PROTEIN: 25G CARB: 15G FAT: 14G FIBER: 5G SUGAR: 1G

INGREDIENTS

2 salmon fillets

2 cups mixed vegetables (such as bell peppers, zucchini, carrots)

2 tablespoons olive oil

1 teaspoon garlic powder

1 teaspoon paprika

Salt and pepper to taste

Lemon wedges for serving

DIRECTIONS

Preheat the oven to 350°F. Arrange the salmon fillets on a baking pan lined with parchment paper.

In a mixing bowl, combine the veggies, olive oil, garlic powder, paprika, salt, and pepper.

Arrange the veggies around the salmon fillets on the baking sheet.

Bake for 15-20 minutes, until the salmon is cooked through and the veggies are soft.

Serve hot, with lemon wedges.

CHICKEN AND RICE SOUP

PREP TIME: 10 MIN COOK TIME: 25MIN TOTAL TIME: 35MIN

SERVINGS: 2

NUTRITIONAL INFORMATION (PER SERVING)
CAL: 250K PROTEIN: 20G CARB: 15G FAT: 5G FIBER: 3G SUGAR: 2G

INGREDIENTS

2 salmon fillets

8 cups chicken broth

2 cups cooked shredded chicken breast

1 cup cooked white rice

2 carrots, diced

2 celery stalks, diced

1 onion, diced

2 cloves garlic, minced

1 teaspoon dried thyme

Salt and pepper to taste

Fresh parsley for garnish

DIRECTIONS

In a large saucepan, bring chicken broth to a simmer over medium heat.

In a saucepan, combine shredded chicken, cooked white rice, chopped carrots, celery, onion, minced garlic, dried thyme, salt, and pepper.

Simmer for 20-25 minutes, until the veggies are soft.

Taste and adjust the seasoning as required.

Serve hot and garnished with fresh parsley.

TURKEY MEATBALLS WITH ZUCCHINI NOODLES

PREP TIME: 15 MIN COOK TIME: 25MIN TOTAL TIME: 40MIN

SERVINGS: 4
NUTRITIONAL INFORMATION (PER SERVING)
CAL: 300K PROTEIN: 25G CARB: 20G FAT: 12G FIBER: 5G SUGAR: 3G

INGREDIENTS

1 pound ground turkey
1/4 cup breadcrumbs
1/4 cup grated Parmesan cheese
1 egg
2 cloves garlic, minced
1 teaspoon Italian seasoning
Salt and pepper to taste
2 large zucchini, spiralized
1 cup marinara sauce
Fresh basil leaves for garnish

DIRECTIONS

Preheat the oven to 375° Fahrenheit (190° Celsius). Line a baking sheet with parchment paper.

In a large mixing bowl, add ground turkey, breadcrumbs, grated Parmesan cheese, egg, chopped garlic, Italian seasoning, salt, and pepper. Mix until well mixed.

Form the mixture into meatballs and put on the prepared baking sheet.

Bake the meatballs for 20-25 minutes, or until well done.

In a pan, cook the marinara sauce over medium heat. Add the spiralized zucchini noodles and cooked meatballs to the skillet.

Cook for 2-3 minutes, until the zucchini noodles are soft.

Serve turkey meatballs and zucchini noodles hot, topped with fresh basil leaves.

QUINOA AND VEGETABLE STIR-FRY

PREP TIME: 15 MIN COOK TIME: 15MIN TOTAL TIME: 30MIN

SERVINGS: 4

NUTRITIONAL INFORMATION (PER SERVING)
CAL: 250K PROTEIN: 10G CARB: 25G FAT: 10G FIBER: 7G SUGAR: 5G

INGREDIENTS

1 cup cooked quinoa

2 cups mixed vegetables (such as bell peppers, broccoli, snap peas)

2 tablespoons soy sauce

1 tablespoon hoisin sauce

1 tablespoon sesame oil

2 cloves garlic, minced

Salt and pepper to taste

Optional: Sliced green onions, sesame seeds for garnish

DIRECTIONS

Heat the sesame oil in a large pan or wok over medium heat.

Sauté the minced garlic for 1 minute.

Stir-fry the mixed veggies in the pan for 5-7 minutes, or until soft and crispy.

Stir in the cooked quinoa, soy sauce, and hoisin sauce. Cook for a further 2-3 minutes.

Taste and adjust seasoning with salt and pepper as required.

Serve hot, topped with chopped green onions and sesame seeds if preferred.

BAKED CHICKEN BREAST WITH SWEET POTATO MASH

PREP TIME: 15 MIN COOK TIME: 25MIN TOTAL TIME: 40MIN

SERVINGS: 2

NUTRITIONAL INFORMATION (PER SERVING)

CAL: 350K PROTEIN: 30G CARB: 25G FAT: 10G FIBER: 5G SUGAR: 4G

INGREDIENTS

2 boneless, skinless chicken breasts

2 medium sweet potatoes, peeled and diced

2 tablespoons olive oil

1 teaspoon garlic powder

1 teaspoon paprika

Salt and pepper to taste

Fresh parsley for garnish

DIRECTIONS

Preheat the oven to 350° F. Place the chicken breasts on a baking pan lined with parchment paper.

Drizzle olive oil over chicken breasts and season with garlic powder, paprika, salt, and pepper.

Bake for 20-25 minutes, until the chicken is fully done and no longer pink in the middle.

While the chicken bakes, cook diced sweet potatoes in a saucepan of water until cooked, approximately 15-20 minutes.

Drain the sweet potatoes and mash with a fork or potato masher until smooth.

Serve baked chicken breasts hot with sweet potato mash, garnished with fresh parsley.

SPAGHETTI SQUASH WITH TOMATO BASIL SAUCE

PREP TIME: 15 MIN COOK TIME: 40MIN TOTAL TIME: 55MIN

SERVINGS: 3

NUTRITIONAL INFORMATION (PER SERVING)

CAL: 200K PROTEIN: 10G CARB: 20G FAT: 8G FIBER: 8G SUGAR: 5G

INGREDIENTS

1 spaghetti squash

2 cups marinara sauce

2 cloves garlic, minced

1/4 cup fresh basil leaves, chopped

Olive oil for drizzling

Salt and pepper to taste

Grated Parmesan cheese for serving

DIRECTIONS

Preheat the oven to 350°F. Cut the spaghetti squash in half lengthwise, then scrape out the seeds.

Place the spaghetti squash halves, cut side down, on a baking sheet lined with parchment paper.

Bake for 30-40 minutes, until the squash is soft and easily punctured with a fork.

While the squash is baking, warm the olive oil in a pan over medium heat. Sauté the minced garlic for 1 minute.

Stir in the marinara sauce and chopped basil leaves. Simmer for 5–10 minutes.

Scrape the flesh of the cooked spaghetti squash with a fork to create spaghetti-like strands.

Serve spaghetti squash topped with tomato basil sauce and grated Parmesan cheese.

GRILLED STEAK WITH ROASTED ASPARAGUS

PREP TIME: 15 MIN COOK TIME: 15MIN TOTAL TIME: 30MIN

SERVINGS: 2

NUTRITIONAL INFORMATION (PER SERVING)

CAL: 400K PROTEIN: 25G CARB: 10G FAT: 25G FIBER: 6G SUGAR: 5G

INGREDIENTS

2 steaks of your choice (such as sirloin, ribeye)

1 pound asparagus spears, trimmed

2 tablespoons olive oil

2 cloves garlic, minced

Salt and pepper to taste

Lemon wedges for serving

DIRECTIONS

Preheat the grill to medium-high heat.

Brush olive oil and minced garlic over steaks and asparagus stalks. Season with salt and pepper.

Grill steaks for 4-5 minutes each side for medium-rare, up to your chosen doneness.

Grill the asparagus spears for 3-4 minutes, rotating periodically, until tender and lightly browned.

Remove the steaks and asparagus from the grill and let them rest for a few minutes.

Grilled steak is served with roasted asparagus and lemon wedges as a garnish.

<u>STUFFED BELL PEPPERS WITH GROUND TURKEY</u>

PREP TIME: 15 MIN COOK TIME: 40MIN TOTAL TIME: 55MIN

SERVINGS: 2

NUTRITIONAL INFORMATION (PER SERVING)
CAL: 300K PROTEIN: 25G CARB: 15G FAT: 15G FIBER: 5G SUGAR: 8G

INGREDIENTS

4 bell peppers, halved and seeds removed
1 pound ground turkey
1 cup cooked quinoa
1 cup marinara sauce
1/2 cup shredded mozzarella cheese
Salt and pepper to taste
Fresh parsley for garnish

DIRECTIONS

Preheat the oven to 375° Fahrenheit (190° Celsius). Place the bell pepper halves in a baking dish.

Cook ground turkey in a skillet until browned. Drain any extra fat.

In a large mixing bowl, add cooked ground turkey, quinoa, marinara sauce, salt, and pepper.

Spoon the turkey and quinoa mixture into each bell pepper half.

Cover the baking dish with foil and bake for 30-35 minutes, until the peppers are soft.

Remove the cover, sprinkle the filled peppers with shredded mozzarella cheese, and bake for another 5 minutes, or until the cheese has melted.

Serve hot, garnished with fresh parsley.

SALMON AND QUINOA SALAD

PREP TIME: 15 MIN COOK TIME: 20 MIN TOTAL TIME: 35MIN

SERVINGS: 2

NUTRITIONAL INFORMATION (PER SERVING)

CAL: 350K PROTEIN: 25G CARB: 15G FAT: 15G FIBER: 8G SUGAR: 5G

INGREDIENTS

2 salmon fillets
1 cup cooked quinoa
4 cups mixed salad greens
Cherry tomatoes, halved
Cucumber, diced
Red onion, thinly sliced
Balsamic vinaigrette dressing

DIRECTIONS

Preheat the oven to 400° F (200° C). Arrange the salmon fillets on a baking pan lined with parchment paper.

Bake the salmon for 15-20 minutes, or until it is well cooked and flaky.

In a large mixing bowl, add the cooked quinoa, mixed salad greens, cherry tomatoes, cucumber, and red onion.

Flake the cooked salmon and add it to the salad.

Toss the salad with the balsamic vinaigrette dressing.

Serve immediately.

<u>VEGETABLE AND LENTIL CURRY</u>

PREP TIME: 15 MIN COOK TIME: 25 MIN TOTAL TIME: 40MIN

SERVINGS: 2

NUTRITIONAL INFORMATION (PER SERVING)
CAL: 300K PROTEIN: 15G CARB: 25G FAT: 10G FIBER: 12G SUGAR: 8G

INGREDIENTS

1 cup lentils, rinsed and drained
2 cups mixed vegetables (such as bell peppers, cauliflower, carrots)
1 onion, chopped
2 cloves garlic, minced
1 can (14 ounces) coconut milk
2 tablespoons curry powder
1 teaspoon ground turmeric
1 teaspoon ground cumin
Salt and pepper to taste
Fresh cilantro for garnish
Cooked rice for serving

DIRECTIONS

In a large saucepan, add lentils, mixed veggies, diced onion, minced garlic,
coconut milk, curry powder, powdered turmeric, ground cumin, salt, and pepper.
Bring to a boil, then decrease the heat and simmer for 20-25 minutes, or until the
lentils and veggies are cooked.
Taste and adjust the seasoning as required.
Serve vegetable and lentil curry hot, topped with fresh cilantro and cooked rice.

SHRIMP AND BROCCOLI STIR-FRY

PREP TIME: 15 MIN COOK TIME: 15 MIN TOTAL TIME: 30MIN

SERVINGS: 2

NUTRITIONAL INFORMATION (PER SERVING)

CAL: 250K PROTEIN: 25G CARB: 15G FAT: 10G FIBER: 5G SUGAR: 5G

INGREDIENTS

8 ounces shrimp, peeled and deveined

2 cups broccoli florets

1 bell pepper, sliced

1 onion, sliced

2 cloves garlic, minced

2 tablespoons soy sauce

1 tablespoon hoisin sauce

1 tablespoon sesame oil

Cooked brown rice for serving

DIRECTIONS

Heat the sesame oil in a large pan or wok over medium heat.

Sauté the minced garlic for 1 minute.

Cook the shrimp in the skillet for 2-3 minutes, until they are pink and fully cooked.

Remove the shrimp from the skillet and put aside.

Add the broccoli florets, sliced bell pepper, and sliced onion to the pan. Stir-fry the veggies for 5-7 minutes, or until soft and crisp.

Return the cooked shrimp to the skillet.

Cook a further 2 minutes after adding the soy sauce and hoisin sauce.

Serve the shrimp and broccoli stir-fry hot with prepared brown rice.

MUSHROOM AND SPINACH RISOTTO

PREP TIME: 15 MIN COOK TIME: 15 MIN TOTAL TIME: 30MIN

SERVINGS: 2

NUTRITIONAL INFORMATION (PER SERVING)

CAL: 350K PROTEIN: 10G CARB: 20G FAT: 10G FIBER: 8G SUGAR: 5G

INGREDIENTS

1 cup Arborio rice

4 cups vegetable broth

1 onion, chopped

2 cloves garlic, minced

8 ounces mushrooms, sliced

2 cups fresh spinach leaves

1/4 cup grated Parmesan cheese

2 tablespoons butter

Salt and pepper to taste

Fresh parsley for garnish

DIRECTIONS

In a saucepan, cook the vegetable broth over medium heat until it simmers.

In a large pan, melt the butter over medium heat. Sauté the chopped onion and minced garlic for 2-3 minutes, until softened.

Cook Arborio rice in the skillet for 1-2 minutes, stirring frequently.

Pour boiling vegetable stock into the pan one ladleful at a time, stirring regularly and letting the liquid soak before adding more.

Continue to add liquid and stir until the rice is creamy and cooked through, approximately 20-25 minutes.

In the final 5 minutes of simmering, add the sliced mushrooms and fresh spinach leaves, stirring until wilted. Remove risotto from the stove and toss in the shredded Parmesan cheese. Season with salt and pepper to taste.

Serve the mushroom and spinach risotto hot, topped with fresh parsley.

<u>EGGPLANT PARMESAN</u>

PREP TIME: 15 MIN COOK TIME: 30 MIN TOTAL TIME: 45MIN

SERVINGS: 4

NUTRITIONAL INFORMATION (PER SERVING)

CAL: 350K PROTEIN: 10G CARB: 20G FAT: 10G FIBER: 8G SUGAR: 5G

INGREDIENTS

large eggplant, sliced into rounds

1 cup marinara sauce

1 cup breadcrumbs

1/4 cup grated Parmesan cheese

1 egg, beaten

1 tablespoon olive oil

Salt and pepper to taste

Fresh basil leaves for garnish

DIRECTIONS

Preheat the oven to 375° Fahrenheit (190° Celsius). Line a baking sheet with parchment paper.

Dip eggplant slices in beaten egg, then cover with breadcrumbs seasoned with grated Parmesan, salt, and pepper.

Place the breaded eggplant slices on the prepared baking sheet.

Drizzle olive oil over the eggplant pieces.

Bake for 25-30 minutes, until the eggplant is soft and the breadcrumbs are golden brown.

Remove from the oven and spread marinara sauce on each eggplant slice.

Return to the oven and bake for another 5 minutes, or until the sauce is well cooked.

Serve eggplant Parmesan hot, topped with fresh basil leaves.

TOFU AND VEGETABLE STIR-FRY

PREP TIME: 15 MIN COOK TIME: 15 MIN TOTAL TIME: 30MIN

SERVINGS: 3

NUTRITIONAL INFORMATION (PER SERVING)

CAL: 250K PROTEIN: 15G CARB: 15G FAT: 12G FIBER: 4G SUGAR: 3G

INGREDIENTS

1 block (14 ounces) extra-firm tofu, pressed and cubed

2 cups mixed vegetables (such as bell peppers, snap peas, carrots)

2 tablespoons soy sauce

1 tablespoon hoisin sauce

1 tablespoon sesame oil

2 cloves garlic, minced

Cooked brown rice for serving

DIRECTIONS

Heat the sesame oil in a large pan or wok over medium heat.

Sauté the minced garlic for 1 minute.

Cook the cubed tofu in the pan until browned on both sides, which should take around 5-7 minutes.

Stir-fry the mixed veggies in the pan for a further 5 minutes, or until tender and crisp.

Cook a further 2 minutes after adding the soy sauce and hoisin sauce.

Serve the tofu and vegetable stir-fry hot with prepared brown rice.

aves.

LEMON HERB GRILLED CHICKEN WITH ROASTED VEGETABLES

PREP TIME: 15 MIN COOK TIME: 15 MIN TOTAL TIME: 30MIN

SERVINGS: 2

NUTRITIONAL INFORMATION (PER SERVING)

CAL: 300K PROTEIN: 30G CARB: 15G FAT: 15G FIBER: 5G SUGAR: 5G

INGREDIENTS

2 chicken breasts

2 cups mixed vegetables (such as bell peppers, zucchini, cherry tomatoes)

2 tablespoons olive oil

2 cloves garlic, minced

Zest and juice of 1 lemon

1 teaspoon dried thyme

1 teaspoon dried rosemary

Salt and pepper to taste

DIRECTIONS

In a mixing bowl, combine olive oil, minced garlic, lemon zest, lemon juice, dried thyme, rosemary, salt, and pepper.

Put the chicken breasts in a shallow dish and pour half of the marinade over them.

Marinate in the refrigerator for a minimum of 30 minutes.

Preheat the grill to medium-high heat.

Thread the mixed veggies on skewers and brush with the leftover marinade.

Grill chicken breasts for 6-8 minutes each side, or until well done and no longer pink in the middle.

Grill the vegetable skewers for 5-7 minutes, rotating periodically, until soft and gently browned.

Serve grilled chicken with roasted veggies.

DESSERT RECIPE

BANANA "NICE" CREAM

PREP TIME: 10 MIN COOK TIME: 5 MIN TOTAL TIME: 15 MIN

SERVINGS: 2

NUTRITIONAL INFORMATION (PER SERVING)

CAL: 100K PROTEIN: 1G   CARB: 30G FAT: 0G FIBER: 5G SUGAR: 10G

INGREDIENTS

2 ripe bananas, sliced and frozen

Optional toppings: chopped nuts, shredded coconut, dark chocolate chips

DIRECTIONS

Place frozen banana slices into a food processor or blender.

Blend until smooth and creamy, scraping down the sides as necessary.

Serve immediately as soft-serve ice cream, or freeze for 1-2 hours for a firmer consistency.

If wanted, top with your favorite toppings.

CHIA SEED PUDDING

PREP TIME: 10 MIN COOK TIME: 5 MIN   TOTAL TIME: 15 MIN

SERVINGS: 2

NUTRITIONAL INFORMATION (PER SERVING)

CAL: 120K PROTEIN: 4G   CARB: 12G FAT: 7G FIBER: 9G SUGAR: 2G

INGREDIENTS

1/4 cup chia seeds

1 cup unsweetened almond milk (or any milk of your choice)

1 tablespoon maple syrup or honey

1/2 teaspoon vanilla extract

Optional toppings: fresh fruit, nuts, seeds

DIRECTIONS

In a bowl, mix together chia seeds, almond milk, maple syrup or honey, and vanilla extract.

Cover and refrigerate for at least 2 hours or overnight, stirring occasionally.

Serve chilled with your favorite toppings.

<u>BAKED APPLES</u>

PREP TIME: 10 MIN COOK TIME: 25 MIN   TOTAL TIME: 15 MIN

SERVINGS: 2

NUTRITIONAL INFORMATION (PER SERVING)

CAL: 100K   PROTEIN: 0G   CARB: 17G FAT: 0G FIBER: 5G SUGAR: 5G

<u>INGREDIENTS</u>

2 apples, cored

2 tablespoons maple syrup or honey

1 teaspoon cinnamon

Optional toppings: Greek yogurt, granola

DIRECTIONS

Preheat the oven to 375° Fahrenheit (190° Celsius).

Place the cored apples onto a baking dish.

Drizzle maple syrup or honey over the apples, then sprinkle with cinnamon.

Bake for 20-25 minutes, until the apples are soft.

Serve warm, with optional toppings as desired.

CHOCOLATE AVOCADO MOUSSE

PREP TIME: 10 MIN COOK TIME: 25 MIN   TOTAL TIME: 15 MIN

SERVINGS: 2

NUTRITIONAL INFORMATION (PER SERVING)

CAL: 200K   PROTEIN: 3G   CARB: 8G   FAT: 14G   FIBER: 7G   SUGAR: 9G

INGREDIENTS

1 ripe avocado

2 tablespoons cocoa powder

2 tablespoons maple syrup or honey

1/2 teaspoon vanilla extract

Pinch of salt

Optional toppings: fresh berries, shredded coconut

DIRECTIONS

Scoop the avocado flesh into a blender or food processor.

Combine cocoa powder, maple syrup or honey, vanilla essence, and a sprinkle of salt.

Blend until smooth and creamy, scraping down the sides as necessary.

Divide into serving dishes and chill for at least 30 minutes before serving.

Top with optional toppings, if desired.

.

<u>COCONUT YOGURT PARFAIT</u>

PREP TIME: 10 MIN COOK TIME: 10 MIN TOTAL TIME: 15 MIN

SERVINGS: 2

NUTRITIONAL INFORMATION (PER SERVING)

CAL: 200K   PROTEIN: 3G   CARB: 18G   FAT: 14G   FIBER: 7G   SUGAR: 9G

<u>INGREDIENTS</u>

1 cup coconut yogurt

1/2 cup granola

1/2 cup mixed berries

Optional toppings: shredded coconut, honey

DIRECTIONS

Layer coconut yogurt, granola, and mixed berries in a serving dish or glass.

Repeat layering until all of the ingredients have been used up.

If desired, add optional toppings.

Serve immediately.

ALMOND BUTTER ENERGY BALLS

PREP TIME: 10 MIN COOK TIME: MIN TOTAL TIME: 40 MIN

SERVINGS: 12 ENERGY BALLS

NUTRITIONAL INFORMATION (PER SERVING)

CAL: 150K   PROTEIN: 5G   CARB: 20G   FAT: 7G   FIBER: 3G   SUGAR: 5G

INGREDIENTS

1 cup rolled oats
1/2 cup almond butter
- 1/4 cup honey
1/4 cup shredded coconut
1/4 cup dark chocolate chips
1 teaspoon vanilla extract
Pinch of salt

DIRECTIONS

In a mixing bowl, add rolled oats, almond butter, honey, shredded coconut, dark chocolate chips, vanilla extract, and a sprinkle of salt until thoroughly blended.
Roll the mixture into little balls with your hands.
Place the energy balls on a baking sheet lined with parchment paper.
Refrigerate for a minimum of 30 minutes before serving.
Serve cold.

FROZEN GRAPES

PREP TIME: 10 MIN COOK TIME: MIN TOTAL TIME: 2 hours 5 MIN

SERVINGS: 2

NUTRITIONAL INFORMATION (PER SERVING)

CAL: 60K   PROTEIN: 1G   CARB: 10G   FAT: 0G   FIBER: 1G   SUGAR: 12G

INGREDIENTS

2 cups grapes (any variety)

DIRECTIONS

Wash grapes and pat them dry with a paper towel.

Place the grapes in a single layer on a baking sheet lined with parchment paper.

Place in the freezer for at least two hours, or until frozen.

Serve frozen grapes as a delightful snack.

RICE CAKE WITH NUT BUTTER AND BANANA

PREP TIME: 10 MIN COOK TIME: 10 MIN TOTAL TIME: 20 MIN

SERVINGS: 2

NUTRITIONAL INFORMATION (PER SERVING)

CAL: 200K   PROTEIN: 5G   CARB: 30G   FAT: 8G   FIBER: 4G   SUGAR: 12G

INGREDIENTS

2 rice cakes

2 tablespoons nut butter (such as almond butter or peanut butter)

1 banana, sliced

DIRECTIONS

Spread nut butter evenly onto rice cakes.

Top with banana slices.

Serve immediately.

GREEK YOGURT WITH HONEY AND NUTS

PREP TIME: 10 MIN COOK TIME: 10 MIN TOTAL TIME: 20 MIN

SERVINGS: 2

NUTRITIONAL INFORMATION (PER SERVING)

CAL: 250K   PROTEIN: 15G   CARB: 20G   FAT: 15G   FIBER: 2G   SUGAR: 10G

INGREDIENTS

1 cup Greek yogurt

2 tablespoons honey

1/4 cup mixed nuts (such as almonds, walnuts, pecans)

DIRECTIONS

In serving dishes, spoon Greek yogurt.

Drizzle with honey.

Sprinkle the mixed nuts on top.

Serve immediately.

BAKED PEARS WITH CINNAMON

PREP TIME: 10 MIN COOK TIME: 25 MIN TOTAL TIME: 35 MIN

SERVINGS: 2

NUTRITIONAL INFORMATION (PER SERVING)

CAL: 100K   PROTEIN: 1G   CARB: 17G   FAT: 0G   FIBER: 5G   SUGAR: 12G

INGREDIENTS

2 pears, halved and cored

1 tablespoon honey

1 teaspoon cinnamon

Optional toppings: Greek yogurt, granola

DIRECTIONS

Preheat the oven to 375° Fahrenheit (190° Celsius).

Place the pear halves in a baking dish.

Drizzle honey over the pears, then sprinkle with cinnamon.

Bake for 20-25 minutes, until the pears are soft.

Serve warm, with optional toppings as desired.

BERRY SMOOTHIE

PREP TIME: 10 MIN COOK TIME: 15 MIN TOTAL TIME: 25 MIN

SERVINGS: 2

NUTRITIONAL INFORMATION (PER SERVING)

CAL: 150K   PROTEIN: 7G   CARB: 26G   FAT: 2G   FIBER: 5G   SUGAR: 15G

INGREDIENTS

1 cup mixed berries (such as strawberries, blueberries, raspberries)

1/2 banana

1/2 cup Greek yogurt

1/2 cup almond milk (or any milk of your choice)

1 tablespoon honey

Ice cubes

DIRECTIONS

In a blender, combine mixed berries, banana, Greek yogurt, almond milk, honey, and ice cubes.

Blend until smooth and creamy.

Serve immediately.

CHOCOLATE COVERED STRAWBERRIES

PREP TIME: 10 MIN COOK TIME: MIN TOTAL TIME: 40 MIN

SERVINGS: 2

NUTRITIONAL INFORMATION (PER SERVING)

CAL: 100K   PROTEIN: 1G   CARB: 15G   FAT: 5G   FIBER: 3G   SUGAR: 10G

INGREDIENTS

1 cup strawberries

1/4 cup dark chocolate chips

DIRECTIONS

Wash strawberries and blot them dry with a paper towel.

Melt dark chocolate chips in a microwave-safe dish at 30-second intervals, stirring in between, until smooth.

Dip each strawberry in melted chocolate, covering approximately halfway.

Place the chocolate-covered strawberries on a baking sheet coated with parchment paper.

Refrigerate for at least 30 minutes until the chocolate has hardened.

Serve cold.

PUMPKIN CHIA SEED PUDDING

PREP TIME: 10 MIN COOK TIME: 15 MIN TOTAL TIME: 2 HOURS

SERVINGS: 2

NUTRITIONAL INFORMATION (PER SERVING)
CAL: 150K   PROTEIN: 5G   CARB: 20G   FAT: 7G   FIBER: 10G   SUGAR: 8G

INGREDIENTS

1/4 cup chia seeds
1 cup unsweetened almond milk (or any milk of your choice)
1/4 cup pumpkin puree
2 tablespoons maple syrup or honey
1/2 teaspoon pumpkin pie spice
Optional toppings: chopped nuts, cinnamon

DIRECTIONS

In a bowl, combine the chia seeds, almond milk, pumpkin puree, maple syrup or honey, and pumpkin pie spice.
Cover and chill for at least 2 hours, preferably overnight, stirring regularly.
Serve cold, with optional toppings.

COCONUT FLOUR PANCAKES

PREP TIME: 10 MIN COOK TIME: MIN TOTAL TIME: 40 MIN

SERVINGS: 2

NUTRITIONAL INFORMATION (PER SERVING)

CAL: 150K   PROTEIN: 7G   CARB: 15G   FAT: 8G   FIBER: 5G   SUGAR: 6G

INGREDIENTS

1/4 cup coconut flour

2 eggs

1/4 cup almond milk (or any milk of your choice)

1 tablespoon maple syrup or honey

1/2 teaspoon baking powder

Pinch of salt

Coconut oil for cooking

Optional toppings: fresh fruit, maple syrup

DIRECTIONS

In a mixing bowl, combine the coconut flour, eggs, almond milk, maple syrup or honey, baking powder, and a sprinkle of salt until smooth.

Heat the coconut oil in a skillet over medium heat.

Pour the pancake batter into the skillet to make little pancakes.

Cook for 2-3 minutes each side, until golden brown and heated through.

Serve heated pancakes with your preferred toppings.

FROZEN BANANA BITES

PREP TIME: 10 MIN COOK TIME: MIN TOTAL TIME1 HOUR 20 MIN

SERVINGS: 4

NUTRITIONAL INFORMATION (PER SERVING)

CAL: 150K   PROTEIN: 3G   CARB: 20G   FAT: 8G   FIBER: 4G   SUGAR: 5G

INGREDIENTS

2 bananas, peeled and sliced into rounds

1/4 cup almond butter

1/4 cup dark chocolate chips

1 tablespoon coconut oil

Optional toppings: shredded coconut, chopped nuts

DIRECTIONS

Place the banana slices on a baking sheet lined with parchment paper.

Spread almond butter on half of the banana slices.

To make sandwiches, top with the leftover banana slices.

In a microwave-safe dish, melt dark chocolate chips and coconut oil for 30 seconds at a time, stirring in between, until smooth.

Dip each banana sandwich in melted chocolate, covering halfway.

Place the chocolate-covered banana bits back onto the baking sheet.

If desired, add optional toppings.

Freeze for at least one hour, or until the chocolate has set.

Serve cold.

VEGETARIAN RECIPE

QUINOA BUDDHA BOWL

PREP TIME: 15 MIN COOK TIME: 20 MIN TOTAL TIME: 35 MIN

SERVINGS: 2

NUTRITIONAL INFORMATION (PER SERVING)

CAL: 400K PROTEIN: 15G   CARB: 22G FAT: 15G FIBER: 12G SUGAR: 5G

INGREDIENTS

1 cup cooked quinoa

1 cup mixed vegetables (such as roasted sweet potatoes, steamed broccoli, sautéed kale)

1/2 cup chickpeas, drained and rinsed

1/4 avocado, sliced

2 tablespoons hummus

1 tablespoon tahini

1 tablespoon lemon juice

Salt and pepper to taste

DIRECTIONS

Divide the cooked quinoa, mixed veggies, and chickpeas into bowls.

Top with avocado slices.

To prepare the dressing, combine hummus, tahini, lemon juice, salt, and pepper in a small mixing dish.

Drizzle dressing over each bowl.

Serve immediately.

VEGAN LENTIL SOUP

PREP TIME: 15 MIN COOK TIME: 30 MIN TOTAL TIME: 45 MIN

SERVINGS: 2

NUTRITIONAL INFORMATION (PER SERVING)

CAL: 250K PROTEIN: 15G   CARB: 10G FAT: 1G FIBER: 15G SUGAR: 5G

INGREDIENTS

1 cup dried lentils, rinsed

4 cups vegetable broth

1 onion, diced

2 carrots, diced

2 celery stalks, diced

2 cloves garlic, minced

1 teaspoon ground cumin

1 teaspoon paprika

Salt and pepper to taste

Fresh parsley for garnish

DIRECTIONS

In a large saucepan, mix together the lentils, vegetable broth, onion, carrots, celery, garlic, cumin, and paprika.

Bring to a boil, then decrease the heat and simmer for 25-30 minutes, or until the lentils are cooked.

Season with salt and pepper to taste.

Serve hot and garnished with fresh parsley.

CHICKPEA SALAD SANDWICH

PREP TIME: 15 MIN COOK TIME: MIN TOTAL TIME: 15 MIN

SERVINGS: 2

NUTRITIONAL INFORMATION (PER SERVING)

CAL: 300K   PROTEIN: 10G   CARB: 10G   FAT: 10G   FIBER: 10G   SUGAR: 5G

INGREDIENTS

1 can chickpeas, drained and rinsed

2 tablespoons vegan mayonnaise

1 tablespoon Dijon mustard

1 stalk celery, finely chopped

1/4 cup red onion, finely chopped

1 tablespoon fresh dill, chopped

Salt and pepper to taste

4 slices whole grain bread

Lettuce, tomato, and avocado for serving

DIRECTIONS

In a bowl, mash chickpeas with a fork until slightly chunky.

Stir in vegan mayonnaise, Dijon mustard, celery, red onion, dill, salt, and pepper.

Toast whole grain bread slices if desired.

Assemble sandwiches with chickpea salad, lettuce, tomato, and avocado.

Serve immediately.

STUFFED BELL PEPPERS

PREP TIME: 15 MIN COOK TIME: 30 MIN TOTAL TIME: 45 MIN

SERVINGS: 2

NUTRITIONAL INFORMATION (PER SERVING)

CAL: 200K PROTEIN: 10G CARB: 16G FAT: 3G FIBER: 10G SUGAR: 5G

INGREDIENTS

4 bell peppers, halved and seeds removed

1 cup cooked quinoa

1 can black beans, drained and rinsed

1 cup corn kernels

1 cup diced tomatoes

1/2 cup diced red onion

1 teaspoon chili powder

1 teaspoon cumin

Salt and pepper to taste

1/2 cup shredded vegan cheese (optional)

Fresh cilantro for garnish

DIRECTIONS

Preheat the oven to 375° Fahrenheit (190° Celsius).

In a large mixing bowl, add cooked quinoa, black beans, corn, diced tomatoes, red onion, chili powder, cumin, salt, and pepper.

Stuff bell pepper halves with the quinoa mixture.

Place the filled bell peppers in a baking dish.

Cover with foil and bake for 25-30 minutes, until the peppers are cooked.

If using vegan cheese, remove the foil and sprinkle it on top of the peppers. Return to the oven and bake for another 5 minutes, or until the cheese has melted.

Garnish with fresh cilantro before serving.

VEGAN CHILI

PREP TIME: 15 MIN COOK TIME: 30 MIN TOTAL TIME: 45 MIN

SERVINGS: 4

NUTRITIONAL INFORMATION (PER SERVING)

CAL: 250K PROTEIN: 10G CARB: 10G FAT: 5G FIBER: 15G SUGAR: 5G

INGREDIENTS

1 tablespoon olive oil

1 onion, diced

2 cloves garlic, minced

1 bell pepper, diced

1 zucchini, diced

1 carrot, diced

1 can diced tomatoes

2 cups vegetable broth

1 can kidney beans, drained and rinsed

1 can black beans, drained and rinsed

1 tablespoon chili powder

1 teaspoon cumin

Salt and pepper to taste and Fresh cilantro for garnish

DIRECTIONS

In a large saucepan, heat the olive oil over medium heat.

Add the diced onion and garlic and cook until tender.

Cook for a further 5 minutes after adding the carrot, zucchini, and bell pepper.

Stir in the chopped tomatoes, vegetable broth, kidney and black beans, chili powder, cumin, salt, and pepper.

Bring to a boil, then cook for 20-25 minutes, stirring regularly.

Adjust the seasoning as required.

Serve hot and topped with fresh cilantro.

<u>SWEET POTATO AND BLACK BEAN TACOS</u>

PREP TIME: 15 MIN COOK TIME: 30 MIN TOTAL TIME: 45 MIN

SERVINGS: 4

NUTRITIONAL INFORMATION (PER SERVING)

CAL: 250K PROTEIN: 8G   CARB: 19G FAT: 5G FIBER: 10G SUGAR: 5G

<u>INGREDIENTS</u>

2 sweet potatoes, peeled and diced

1 tablespoon olive oil

1 teaspoon chili powder

1 teaspoon cumin

Salt and pepper to taste

1 can black beans, drained and rinsed

8 small corn tortillas

Toppings: avocado slices, shredded lettuce, diced tomatoes, salsa, lime wedges

DIRECTIONS

Preheat the oven to 400° F (200° C).

In a mixing dish, combine the diced sweet potatoes, olive oil, chili powder, cumin, salt, and pepper.

Spread the sweet potatoes in a single layer on a baking pan.

Roast in the oven for 20-25 minutes, until soft and gently browned.

Heat black beans in a small saucepan over medium heat until they are warmed through.

Warm corn tortillas on a dry skillet or in the microwave.

Fill tacos with roasted sweet potatoes, black beans, and any preferred toppings.

Serve immediately with lime wedges.

VEGAN STIR-FRY

PREP TIME: 15 MIN COOK TIME: 10 MIN TOTAL TIME: 35 MIN

SERVINGS: 4

NUTRITIONAL INFORMATION (PER SERVING)

CAL: 150K   PROTEIN: 5G   CARB: 11G   FAT: 7G   FIBER: 7G   SUGAR: 5G

INGREDIENTS

2 tablespoons sesame oil

1 onion, sliced

2 cloves garlic, minced

1 bell pepper, sliced

1 cup broccoli florets

1 cup sliced mushrooms

1 cup snap peas

1 carrot, sliced

1/4 cup soy sauce

1 tablespoon rice vinegar

1 tablespoon maple syrup

1 tablespoon cornstarch. Cooked rice or noodles for serving

DIRECTIONS

In a large skillet or wok, heat the sesame oil over medium-high.

Sauté sliced onion and chopped garlic until tender.

In the pan, combine the sliced bell pepper, broccoli florets, sliced mushrooms, snap peas, and carrot.

Cook for 5-7 minutes, stirring regularly, until the veggies are soft and crisp.

In a small bowl, combine the soy sauce, rice vinegar, maple syrup, and cornstarch.

Pour the sauce over the veggies in the pan, stirring to incorporate. Cook for a further 2-3 minutes, or until the sauce thickens.

Serve hot with prepared rice or noodles.

VEGAN PASTA PRIMAVERA

PREP TIME: 15 MIN COOK TIME: 15 MIN TOTAL TIME: 30 MIN
SERVINGS: 4

NUTRITIONAL INFORMATION (PER SERVING)

CAL: 250K PROTEIN: 8G CARB: 21G FAT: 7G FIBER: 8G SUGAR: 8G

INGREDIENTS

8 ounces whole wheat pasta

2 tablespoons olive oil

2 cloves garlic, minced

1 onion, diced

1 bell pepper, thinly sliced

1 zucchini, thinly sliced

1 yellow squash, thinly sliced

1 cup cherry tomatoes, halved

1 cup baby spinach

1/4 cup chopped fresh basil

Salt and pepper to taste

Vegan parmesan cheese for serving (optional)

DIRECTIONS

Cook the pasta according to package directions until al dente. Drain and put aside.

In a large skillet, heat the olive oil over medium heat.

Sauté minced garlic and sliced onion until softened.

Cook the sliced bell pepper, zucchini, and yellow squash in the pan for about 5-7 minutes, or until soft.

Stir in the cherry tomatoes, baby spinach, and cooked pasta.

Cook for a further 2-3 minutes, until the spinach wilts and the tomatoes soften.

Season with salt and pepper to taste, then top with chopped fresh basil.

Serve hot, with optional vegan parmesan cheese.

<u>CAULIFLOWER RICE STIR-FRY</u>

PREP TIME: 15 MIN COOK TIME: 15 MIN TOTAL TIME: 30 MIN

SERVINGS: 4

NUTRITIONAL INFORMATION (PER SERVING)

CAL: 150K   PROTEIN: 5G   CARB: 20G   FAT: 7G   FIBER: 8G   SUGAR: 8G

<u>INGREDIENTS</u>

1 head cauliflower, riced

2 tablespoons sesame oil

2 cloves garlic, minced

1 onion, diced

1 bell pepper, thinly sliced

1 cup chopped broccoli

1 cup sliced mushrooms

1 cup shredded carrots

1/4 cup soy sauce

1 tablespoon rice vinegar

1 tablespoon maple syrup

Cooked edamame or tofu for serving (optional)

DIRECTIONS

To rice cauliflower, cut it into florets and pulse in a food processor until it resembles rice.

In a large skillet or wok, heat the sesame oil over medium-high.

Sauté minced garlic and sliced onion until softened.

Add thinly sliced bell pepper, chopped broccoli, sliced mushrooms, and shredded carrots to the pan. Cook for 5-7 minutes, stirring regularly, until the veggies are soft and crisp. Stir in the rice cauliflower and simmer for another 2-3 minutes.

In a small bowl, combine the soy sauce, rice vinegar, and maple syrup.

Pour the sauce over the cauliflower mixture in the pan and stir until combined.

Cook for a further 2-3 minutes, or until the sauce thickens.

Serve hot, with cooked edamame or tofu if desired.

<u>VEGAN LENTIL CURRY</u>

PREP TIME: 15 MIN COOK TIME: 30 MIN TOTAL TIME: 45 MIN

SERVINGS: 4

NUTRITIONAL INFORMATION (PER SERVING)

CAL: 300K PROTEIN: 15G CARB: 40G FAT: 10G FIBER: 15G SUGAR: 5G

<u>INGREDIENTS</u>

1 tablespoon coconut oil

1 onion, diced

2 cloves garlic, minced

1 tablespoon grated ginger

1 tablespoon curry powder

1 teaspoon ground cumin

1 teaspoon ground coriander

1/2 teaspoon turmeric

1 cup dried green lentils, rinsed

4 cups vegetable broth

1 can coconut milk

2 cups diced tomatoes

2 cups chopped spinach

Salt and pepper to taste

Cooked rice for serving

DIRECTIONS

In a big saucepan, heat the coconut oil over medium heat. Sauté chopped onion, minced garlic, and grated ginger until softened.Cook for another minute, stirring in curry powder, powdered cumin, ground coriander, and turmeric until aromatic. Add the rinsed green lentils, vegetable broth, coconut milk, and chopped tomatoes to the saucepan. Bring to a boil, then decrease the heat and simmer for 20-25 minutes, or until the lentils are cooked. Stir in the chopped spinach and simmer until wilted. Season with salt and pepper to taste. Serve hot with prepared rice.

VEGAN BURRITO BOWL

PREP TIME: 15 MIN   COOK TIME: 10MIN TOTAL TIME: 25 MIN

SERVINGS: 2

NUTRITIONAL INFORMATION (PER SERVING)

CAL: 300K   PROTEIN: 10G   CARB: 17G   FAT: 10G   FIBER: 15G   SUGAR: 5G

INGREDIENTS

1 cup cooked quinoa

1 can black beans, drained and rinsed

1 cup corn kernels

1 cup diced tomatoes

1/2 cup diced red onion

1/4 cup chopped fresh cilantro

1 avocado, sliced

Juice of 1 lime

Salt and pepper to taste

DIRECTIONS

In a bowl, add cooked quinoa, black beans, corn kernels, diced tomatoes, red onion, and cilantro.

Toss the ingredients with the squeezed lime juice.

Season with salt and pepper to taste.

Divide the quinoa mixture into bowls and top with sliced avocado.

Serve immediately.

CHICKPEA AND SPINACH COCONUT CURRY

PREP TIME: 15 MIN   COOK TIME: 20 MIN TOTAL TIME: 35 MIN

SERVINGS: 4

NUTRITIONAL INFORMATION (PER SERVING)

CAL: 300K   PROTEIN: 10G   CARB: 14G   FAT: 15G   FIBER: 10G   SUGAR: 5G

INGREDIENTS

1 tablespoon coconut oil

1 onion, diced

2 cloves garlic, minced

1 tablespoon grated ginger

1 tablespoon curry powder

1 teaspoon ground cumin

1 teaspoon ground coriander

1/2 teaspoon turmeric

1 can chickpeas, drained and rinsed

1 can diced tomatoes

1 can coconut milk

2 cups chopped spinach

Salt and pepper to taste

Cooked rice for serving

DIRECTIONS

In a large pan, heat the coconut oil over medium heat. Sauté chopped onion, minced garlic, and grated ginger until softened. Cook for another minute, stirring in curry powder, powdered cumin, ground coriander, and turmeric until aromatic. Add the chickpeas, chopped tomatoes, and coconut milk to the skillet. Bring to a boil, then cook for 10-15 minutes, stirring regularly. Stir in the chopped spinach and simmer until wilted. Season with salt and pepper to taste. Serve hot with prepared rice.

VEGAN LENTIL SHEPHERD'S PIE

PREP TIME: 15 MIN   COOK TIME: 30 MIN TOTAL TIME: 45 MIN

SERVINGS: 4

NUTRITIONAL INFORMATION (PER SERVING)

CAL: 300K   PROTEIN: 10G   CARB: 10G FAT: 10G FIBER: 15G SUGAR: 5G

INGREDIENTS

2 cups cooked lentils

1 onion, diced

2 carrots, diced

2 celery stalks, diced

2 cloves garlic, minced

1 cup vegetable broth

2 tablespoons tomato paste

1 teaspoon thyme

1 teaspoon rosemary

Salt and pepper to taste

4 cups mashed potatoes

Fresh parsley for garnish

DIRECTIONS

Preheat the oven to 375° Fahrenheit (190° Celsius).

In a large pan, cook the chopped onion, carrots, celery, and garlic until softened.

Add the cooked lentils, vegetable broth, tomato paste, thyme, rosemary, salt, and pepper to the skillet. Stir to incorporate, then boil for 10-15 minutes, or until thickened. Transfer the lentil mixture to a baking dish.

Spread the mashed potatoes evenly over the lentil mixture.

Bake in a preheated oven for 25-30 minutes, until golden brown.

Garnish with fresh parsley before serving.

VEGAN PAD THAI

PREP TIME: 15 MIN   COOK TIME: 15 MIN TOTAL TIME: 30 MIN
SERVINGS: 4
NUTRITIONAL INFORMATION (PER SERVING)
CAL: 310K   PROTEIN: 15G   CARB: 15G   FAT: 10G   FIBER: 5G   SUGAR: 10G

INGREDIENTS

8 ounces rice noodles
2 tablespoons soy sauce
2 tablespoons maple syrup
1 tablespoon rice vinegar
1 tablespoon lime juice
1 tablespoon sesame oil
2 cloves garlic, minced
1 shallot, minced
1 cup diced tofu
1 cup shredded carrots
1 cup bean sprouts
1/4 cup chopped peanuts
Fresh cilantro for garnish

DIRECTIONS

Cook the rice noodles according to the package directions.

In a small mixing bowl, combine soy sauce, maple syrup, rice vinegar, lime juice, and sesame oil to create the sauce.

In a large skillet or wok, heat the olive oil over medium heat.

Sauté minced garlic and shallot until softened.

Cook the cubed tofu until it is gently browned.

Stir in the shredded carrots and bean sprouts, and simmer for another 2-3 minutes.

Toss the cooked rice noodles and sauce in the skillet until well combined.

Cook for a another 2-3 minutes, or until heated through.

Serve hot, topped with chopped peanuts and fresh cilantro.

VEGAN EGGPLANT PARMESAN

PREP TIME: 15 MIN   COOK TIME: 35 MIN TOTAL TIME: 50 MIN

SERVINGS: 4

NUTRITIONAL INFORMATION (PER SERVING)

CAL: 250K   PROTEIN: 8G   CARB: 10G   FAT: 10G   FIBER: 10G   SUGAR: 10G

INGREDIENTS

2 eggplants, sliced into rounds

1 cup almond flour

1 teaspoon garlic powder

1 teaspoon dried oregano

Salt and pepper to taste

1 cup marinara sauce

1 cup vegan mozzarella cheese

Fresh basil for garnish

DIRECTIONS

Preheat the oven to 375° Fahrenheit (190° Celsius).

In a small bowl, mix together almond flour, garlic powder, dried oregano, salt, and pepper.

Dredge eggplant slices in the almond flour mixture and shake off any excess.

Place the oiled eggplant slices on a baking sheet lined with parchment paper.

Bake in a preheated oven for 20-25 minutes, or until golden brown and crisp.

Remove from the oven and apply marinara sauce on each eggplant slice.

Sprinkle the vegan mozzarella cheese on top.

Return to the oven and cook for another 10-15 minutes, or until the cheese is melted and bubbling.

Garnish with fresh basil before serving.

DINING OUT AND TRAVELING

Dining Out: Before eating out, research places in advance to find ones that offer Crohn's-friendly choices such as grilled meats, steamed veggies, and simple preparations. Look for meals online and read reviews from other guests. When eating out, don't hesitate to explain your food needs and tastes to restaurant staff. Ask questions about menu items, food replacements, and cooking methods to ensure they match with your dietary limits. Don't be afraid to adjust your order to make it more Crohn's-friendly.

Ask for sauces and dressings on the side, request steamed or grilled choices instead of fried, and replace high-fiber sides with easier-to-digest alternatives. Pay attention to serving sizes when eating out, as big meals can be stressful for your digestive system. Consider getting starters or sharing meals with dinner partners to control serving sizes.

Avoid Trigger Foods: Be aware of trigger foods that may worsen your symptoms, such as hot foods, high-fat meals, and dairy products. Choose food items that are easy on your digestive system and less likely to cause pain. Drink plenty of water while eating out to stay refreshed and support gut health. Avoid sugary drinks and excessive booze, as they can worsen symptoms and add to dehydration.

Traveling: Bring Crohn's-friendly snacks with you when moving to ensure you have healthy options on hand. Pack items such as nuts, seeds, nut butter packs, dried fruits, rice cakes, and low-fiber granola bars for easy and handy snacks. Research food options at your travel spot before your trip to find places and shopping shops that offer Crohn's-friendly choices. Look for rooms with kitchenettes or mini-fridges to store fresh things.

Plan your meals and snacks in advance while moving to avoid depending on new or possibly trigger foods. Consider taking a small cooler with perishable items or bringing a compact mixer for making drinks on the go. Drink plenty of water while moving to stay refreshed and support gut health. Bring a portable water bottle with you and refill it regularly, especially in hot or sticky areas.

HOW TO PLAN FOR TRAVEL WITH CROHN'S DISEASE

Planning for travel with Crohn's disease includes careful planning to ensure that you have everything you need to handle your condition while away from home. Here are some tips to help you plan for travel with Crohn's disease:

Consult Your Healthcare Provider: Before going, schedule a meeting with your healthcare provider to talk your trip plans and ensure that you are in good health to travel. Your healthcare source can also provide advice on handling your condition while away from home and give any necessary medicines or supplies.

Pack an Emergency Kit: Pack a travel-sized emergency kit holding important medications, including prescription medications, over-the-counter treatments for diarrhea and stomach pain, and any other drugs you may need. Also include things such as hand lotion, wet wipes, and throwaway gloves for cleaning reasons. Don't forget to pack supplements you may need while traveling, including prescription medications, over-the-counter treatments. Pay attention to how your body acts to different foods and surroundings while moving. If you notice any signs or pain, take a break, rest, and promote self-care.

Carry Necessary Documentation: Carry a copy of your medical papers, including a list of your current medicines, any allergies or food limits, and contact information for your healthcare provider. This information can be helpful in case of a medical emergency or if you need to seek medical care while abroad. Research healthcare facilities at your destination in advance, including hospitals, clinics, and pharmacists. Familiarize yourself with their sites and contact information so that you know where to go in case of a medical emergency. Pack a sufficient stock of any medical supplies you may need, such as, ostomy supplies, and food vitamins. It's better to have more than you think you'll need to avoid running out while moving.

Stay refreshed: Stay refreshed while flying by drinking plenty of water throughout your trip. Dehydration can exacerbate signs of Crohn's disease, so it's important to drink enough water, especially if you're flying or going to a warm environment. Plan your meals and snacks in advance to ensure that you have access to Crohn's-friendly options while traveling. Research places and shopping stores at your destination that offer reasonable options, and consider taking your own snacks for times when food choices may be limited.

Choose Accommodations Wisely: Choose accommodations that are comfortable and easy for controlling your health. Consider factors such as access to bathroom facilities, closeness to healthcare facilities, and features such as a refrigerator or kitchenette for keeping and making Crohn's-friendly meals.

LIFESTYLE CONSIDERATIONS

STRESS MANAGEMENT TECHNIQUES:

Managing stress is important for people with Crohn's disease, as stress can worsen symptoms and negatively impact general well-being. Here are some stress control methods that can help people with Crohn's disease:

Deep Breathing: Practice deep breathing techniques to promote calm and lower stress. Sit or lie down in a comfortable position, close your eyes, and take slow, deep breaths, focused on filling your belly with air. Hold each breath for a few seconds before releasing slowly. Repeat this process for several minutes to calm your thoughts and body.

Mindfulness Meditation: Engage in mindfulness meditation to develop present-moment focus and lower stress. Find a quiet place where you won't be bothered, sit easily, and focus your mind on your breath or a specific item. Notice any thoughts, feelings, or sensations that come without judgment, and gently guide your focus back to the present moment whenever your mind wanders.

Progressive Muscle Relaxation: Practice progressive muscle relaxation to release stress and promote calm throughout your body. Start by tensing and then releasing each muscle group, starting from your toes and making your way up to your head. Focus on the feelings of tightness and release in each muscle group, allowing yourself to let go of worry and strain with each breath.

Exercise Regularly: Engage in regular physical movement to lower stress and improve general well-being. Choose things that you enjoy, such as walks, swimming, yoga, or tai chi, and aim for at least 30 minutes of mild exercise most days of the week. Exercise releases endorphins, which are natural mood lifters that can help relieve stress and improve mood.

Maintain a Healthy Lifestyle: Prioritize self-care tasks that support physical and mental well-being, such as getting adequate sleep, eating a balanced diet, staying hydrated, and avoiding excessive alcohol and coffee. Taking care of your body and mind can help you better cope with stress and handle your Crohn's disease effectively.

Seek Support: Reach out to friends, family members, or support groups for mental support and guidance. Sharing your experiences with others who understand what you're going through can help you feel less isolated and more supported in controlling your condition.

Practice Time Management: Manage your time successfully to reduce worry and overload. Break tasks down into smaller, doable steps, organize your responsibilities, and share tasks when possible. Set realistic goals and dates for yourself, and be open in changing your plans as needed.
Limit Exposure to Stressful Situations: Identify and lessen causes of stress in your life, whether they're connected to work, relationships, or other areas of your life. Set limits to protect your time and energy, and avoid scenarios or people that cause worry whenever possible.

Engage in Relaxing Activities: Make time for activities that help you relax and unwind, such as reading, listening to music, spending time in nature, or practicing skills and interests. Doing things that bring you joy and relaxation can help lower stress and improve your general quality of life.
Consider Professional Help: If you're fighting to handle stress on your own, consider getting help from a mental health professional such as a therapist or psychologist. They can provide you with additional coping techniques, help, and advice suited to your unique needs.

EXERCISE AND PHYSICAL ACTIVITY RECOMMENDATIONS

Exercise and physical exercise play an important part in controlling Crohn's disease by boosting general health, lowering inflammation, and improving mood and energy levels. Here are some fitness and physical movement suggestions for people with Crohn's disease:

Check Your Healthcare Provider: Before starting any exercise program, check with your healthcare provider to ensure that it's safe and appropriate for your individual situation. They can provide advice on the types and levels of exercise that are good for you.
Start Slowly: If you're new to exercise or have been idle for a while, start slowly and gradually increase the volume and length of your workouts. Begin with low-impact activities such as walking, swimming, or riding, and gradually add more difficult routines as your fitness level improves.

Choose Low-Impact Activities: Opt for low-impact activities that are gentle on the joints and digestive system, especially if you experience stomach pain or soreness. Swimming, riding, yoga, tai chi, and walking are all excellent choices for people with Crohn's disease.

Focus on Flexibility and Strength: Incorporate flexibility and strength training techniques into your practice to improve movement, stability, and muscle power. Pilates, yoga, and manual movements such as squats, lunges, and dips can help strengthen the core muscles and improve general health.

Stay Hydrated: Drink plenty of water before, during, and after exercise to stay hydrated and support digestion. Dehydration can exacerbate symptoms and increase the risk of problems, so it's important to drink enough fluids, especially during hard workouts or in hot weather.

Be Consistent: Aim for stability in your exercise practice by booking regular workouts throughout the week. Even small bouts of exercise can have benefits, so try to add physical movement into your daily routine whenever possible.
Warm Up and Cool Down: Always warm up before exercise and cool down later to avoid harm and ease muscle soreness. Spend a few minutes doing active stretches or light jogging before your workout, and finish with motionless stretches to improve flexibility and promote rest.

Consider Professional Guidance: If you're unsure about how to safely and effectively exercise with Crohn's disease, consider working with a trained fitness trainer or physical therapist who has experience working with people with chronic illnesses. They can provide personalized advice and support to help you meet your exercise goals while controlling your condition effectively.

CONCLUSION

FINAL WORDS OF ENCOURAGEMENT

In conclusion, living with Crohn's disease offers unique hurdles, but it's important to remember that you are not alone. With the right help, tools, and tactics, you can effectively control your situation and lead a happy life.

Remember to value self-care, listen to your body, and fight for your needs. Surround yourself with a caring network of family, friends, healthcare workers, and fellow people dealing with Crohn's disease.

Stay aware about your situation, continue to educate yourself, and try different treatment choices that work best for you. Embrace a healthy lifestyle, including a good diet, regular exercise, stress management methods, and adequate rest.

Above all, be kind to yourself and enjoy your wins, no matter how small. Living with Crohn's disease takes grit, guts, and determination, and you are stronger than you think. Keep moving forward, stay upbeat, and never lose hope. You've got this!

ACKNOWLEDGMENTS

In creating this thorough guide, we'd like to show our thanks to the following people and organizations:

Healthcare Providers: Thank you to the doctors, nurses, and healthcare workers who provide expert care, advice, and support to people living with Crohn's disease. Patients and Caregivers: A sincere thank you to all the patients and caregivers who freely share their experiences, insights, and knowledge, helping to build a helpful community and fostering understanding and empathy.

We offer our thanks to the Crohn's & Colitis Foundation for their commitment to better the lives of people touched by Crohn's disease and ulcerative colitis through study, lobbying, and support services.

Authors and Experts: Thank you to the authors, researchers, and experts whose important contributions to the field of gastroenterology and inflammatory bowel disease have improved our understanding of Crohn's disease and informed the content of this guide.

Support Groups and Online Communities: We realize the importance of support groups and online communities in offering motivation, connection, and tools to people living with Crohn's disease. Your efforts are truly priceless.
Family and Friends: Last but not least, we show our greatest thanks to the family members, friends, and loved ones who offer constant support, understanding, and guidance to those living with Crohn's disease. Your love and kindness make all the difference.

Together, we are joined in our goal to raise awareness, promote education, and help people living with Crohn's disease on their road to better health and well-being. Thank you to everyone who adds to making a good change in the lives of those touched by this situation.

<u>Notes</u>